Current Cardiovascular Therapy

Series Editor
Juan Carlos Kaski

Karen Sliwa • John Anthony
Editors

Cardiac Drugs in Pregnancy

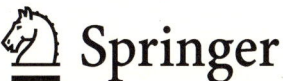 Springer

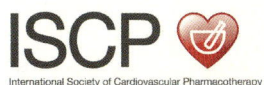

Editors

Karen Sliwa
Department of Medicine,
Faculty of Health Sciences
Hatter Institute for
Cardiovascular Research
in Africa
Cape Town
Western Cape
South Africa

John Anthony
Department of Obstetrics
and Gynaecology
Groote Schuur Hospital
Cape Town
South Africa

ISBN 978-1-4471-5471-6   ISBN 978-1-4471-5472-3   (eBook)
DOI 10.1007/978-1-4471-5472-3
Springer London Heidelberg New York Dordrecht

Library of Congress Control Number: 2013954833

Printed on acid-free paper

Springer is part of Springer Science+Business Media (www.springer.com)

Preface

The spectrum of cardiovascular disease affecting women in pregnancy and postpartum is changing and differs between countries. In the western world, the risk of cardiovascular disease in pregnancy has increased due to the increasing age at the first pregnancy and the worldwide obesity epidemic leading also to early diabetes and hypertension. In addition, the treatment of congenital heart disease has improved leading to an increased number of women with residual heart disease reaching childbearing age. In the western world maternal heart disease is now the major cause of maternal death during pregnancy. In the developing world rheumatic heart disease and the cardiomyopathies dominate. Those women often need anticoagulation as they might have had a valve replacement or formed a thrombus in the left heart. Drugs during pregnancy and the breastfeeding period is a complex subject and there is a profound shortage of evidence based recommendations. As drug treatment in pregnancy concern the mother and the fetus, optimum treatment of both must be targeted.

This book aims at discussing the most important indications of drug usage in pregnancy and postpartum with the aim of weighing the potential risk of a drug and the possible benefit against each other.

Cape Town, South Africa   Karen Sliwa
Cape Town, South Africa   John Anthony

Series Preface

Cardiovascular pharmacotherapy is of fundamental importance for the successful management of patients with cardiovascular diseases. Appropriate therapeutic decisions require a proper understanding of the disease and a thorough knowledge of the pharmacological agents available for clinical use. The issue is complicated by the existence of large numbers of agents with subtle differences in their mode of action and efficacy and the existence of national and international guidelines, which sometimes fail to deliver a clear-cut message. Aggressive marketing techniques from pharma industry; financial issues at local, regional, or national levels; and time constraints make it difficult for the practitioner to – at times – be absolutely certain as to whether drug selection is absolutely appropriate. The International Society of Cardiovascular Pharmacotherapy (ISCP) aims at supporting evidence-based, rational pharmacotherapy worldwide. This book series represents one of its vital educational tools. The books in this series aim at contributing independent, balanced, and sound information to help the busy practitioner to identify the appropriate pharmacological tools and to deliver rational therapies. Topics in the series include all major cardiovascular scenarios, and the books are edited and authored by experts in their fields. The books are intended for a wide range of healthcare professionals and particularly for younger consultants and physicians in training. All aspects of pharmacotherapy are tackled in the series in a concise and practical fashion. The books in this series provide a unique set of guidelines and examples that will prove valuable for patient management. They clearly articulate many of the dilemmas clinicians face when working to deliver sound therapies to their patients. The series will most certainly be a useful reference for those seeking to deliver evidence-based, practical, and successful cardiovascular pharmacotherapy.

Juan Carlos Kaski, DSc, DM (Hons),
MD, FRCP, FESC, FACC, FAHA,
ISCP Current Cardiovascular Therapy Series

Contents

Contributors

John Anthony, MB, ChB, FCOG, MPhil Department of Obstetrics and Gynaecology, Groote Schuur Hospital, Cape Town, South Africa

Eckhart J. Buchmann, MBBCh, FCOG (SA), MSc (Epidemiology), PhD Department of Obstetrics and Gynaecology, University of the Witwatersrand, Johannesburg, South Africa

Catherine Elliott, MBChB, FCOG (SA), MMED (UCT) Department of Obstetrics and Gynaecology, Groote Schuur Hospital, Cape Town, South Africa

Christa Gohlke-Baerwolf, MD Department of Cardiology, Heart Center Bad Krozingen, Krozingen, Germany

Bernard Iung, MD Cardiology Department, AP-HP, Bichat Hospital Paris, Paris, France

University Paris Diderot, Sorbonne Paris Cité, Paris, France

Petronella G. Pieper, MD Department of Cardiology, University Medical Center Groningen, University of Groningen, Groningen, The Netherlands

Vera Regitz-Zagrosek, MD Charité, University Medicine Berlin, Institute of Gender in Medicine (GiM), Berlin, Germany

University Medicine Berlin, Center for Cardiovascular Research (CCR), Berlin, Germany

Jolien W. Roos-Hesselink, MD, PhD Department of Cardiology, Thorax Center, Erasmus Medical Center, Rotterdam, The Netherlands

Titia P.E. Ruys, MD Department of Cardiology, Thorax Center, Erasmus Medical Center, Rotterdam, The Netherlands

Karen Sliwa, MD, PhD, FESC, FACC Department of Medicine, Faculty of Health Sciences, Hatter Institute for Cardiovascular Research in Africa, Groote Schuur Hospital & University of Cape Town, Cape Town, South Africa

Soweto Cardiovascular Research Unit, Chris Hani Baragwanath Hospital, University of the Witwatersrand, Johannesburg, South Africa

Kemilembe B. Tibazarwa, MD, MPH Department of Medicine, Faculty of Health Sciences, Hatter Institute for Cardiovascular Research in Africa, Groote Schuur Hospital & University of Cape Town, Cape Town, South Africa

Soweto Cardiovascular Research Unit, Chris Hani Baragwanath Hospital, University of the Witwatersrand, Johannesburg, South Africa

Annemien E. van den Bosch, MD, PhD Department of Cardiology, Thorax center, Erasmus Medical Center, Rotterdam, The Netherlands

General Principles and Guidelines

John Anthony

Drugs are commonly taken during pregnancy, both by prescription and as over the counter medication. Drugs used during pregnancy may show an altered pharmacodynamic profile when compared to their use in the non-pregnant population. In addition, they may cross the placenta and result in adverse effects on the fetus. There are relatively few data outlining the pharmacodynamic changes characteristic of pregnancy and new drugs are seldom tested in pregnancy when clinical trials are instituted. Prescribing drugs in pregnancy necessarily requires some knowledge of how the pregnancy may alter the pharmacodynamic profile of individual agents and a consideration of any potential adverse effects on the fetus. The use of prescription drugs can only be justified when the anticipated benefits outweigh any known risk. Prescription drugs will be needed in the management of cardiac disease and an understanding of pregnancy physiology will assist in assessing the likely efficacy and risks of these drugs.

J. Anthony, MB, ChB, FCOG, MPhil
Department of Obstetrics and Gynaecology, Groote Schuur Hospital, Observatory, Cape Town 7925, South Africa
e-mail: john.anthony@uct.ac.za

K. Sliwa, J. Anthony (eds.), *Cardiac Drugs in Pregnancy*,
Current Cardiovascular Therapy,
DOI 10.1007/978-1-4471-5472-3_1,
© Springer-Verlag London 2014

Pregnancy Physiology and Pharmacodynamics

The physiological adaptation to pregnancy can affect the absorption, distribution, metabolism and excretion of drugs resulting in sub-therapeutic treatment in some circumstances. The physiological adaptation to pregnancy cannot be simply summated when trying to anticipate the extent to which the non-pregnant pharmacodynamic and pharmacotherapeutic profiles shift during pregnancy. Complex changes may be found in enzyme induction and metabolism, protein binding and excretory function (Isoherranen and Thummel 2013; Anderson 2005). The pregnancy physiology may be transformed by co-morbidity due to illness, the effects of which have been even less studied than pregnancy itself. Finally, the potential exposure of the fetus to drugs may lead to teratogenic as well as other adverse consequences in the neonatal period.

Notwithstanding the deficit in our understanding regarding pharmacodynamic and therapeutic changes of pregnancy, some knowledge about the physiological changes of pregnancy may alert the clinician to potential problems when prescribing drugs during pregnancy.

Physiological Adaptation to Pregnancy and the Cardiovascular System

Increased Plasma Volume

During pregnancy the plasma volume increases by up to 45 % above non-pregnant values, with a net increase of about 1.2 l reached at 30–34 weeks (Sibai and Frangieh 1995). This increase is attained by means of physiological hyperaldosteronism, stimulating renal retention of sodium and water. The retention of water by pregnant women is not confined to the intravascular compartment with dependent interstitial oedema developing towards the end of pregnancy. These increases in intra and extravascular volume have adaptive importance related, firstly, to the necessary increase in cardiac output which ensures an increased rate of delivery of oxygenated blood to the peripheral tissues including the uterus. Fetal oxygenation is thus dependent on volume expansion and increased cardiac output. The increased extra-vascular volume allows physiological protection against haemorrhage during childbirth by creating an extravascular reservoir of fluid that can be redistributed into the intravas-cular compartment should haemorrhage develop following delivery. This increase in intra and extravascular volume cre-ates a larger volume of distribution for drugs administered during pregnancy and non-pregnancy dosing regimens may thus give rise to sub-therapeutic serum concentrations.

Increased Cardiac Output

Cardiac output rises during pregnancy by 30–50 %, beginning from early pregnancy and is maintained throughout preg-nancy (Mabie et al. 1994). The early rise in cardiac output is dependent on an increase in pulse rate with the subsequent volume expansion allowing a rise in stroke volume to sustain the increased cardiac output toward the end of the pregnancy. The slight decline in cardiac output sometimes described toward the end of pregnancy has been attributed to the pos-tural effects of caval compression by the gravid uterus. These changes in cardiac output ensure accelerated delivery of oxy-genated blood to all peripheral organs, the most significant change amongst which is enhanced uterine perfusion. The consequences of increased cardiac output are manifest when arteriovenous oxygen difference is measured by assessing both peripheral arterial oxygen concentration and mixed venous oxygen concentration (acquired by sampling right atrial blood). This measurement demonstrates a reduction in the difference between arteriovenous oxygen concentration for most of pregnancy despite the extra metabolic demands made by the pregnancy (de Swiet 1980). The arteriovenous gap widens towards non-pregnancy levels as the pregnancy approaches term indicating the increasing metabolic demands of the rapidly growing fetus. It is notable that this measurement is a good indication of how the pregnancy adaptation precedes and exceeds the physiological demands of pregnancy for much of the pregnancy. With regard to vasoactive drug therapy, those agents that limit volume expansion or decrease cardiac output may be expected to have an effect on this mechanism. Having an effect on one aspect of the physiological change of pregnancy may not lead to a measurably adverse outcome because the pregnancy adaptation extends beyond the requirements of normal pregnancy.

Vasodilatation

The increased blood volume and cardiac output of normal pregnancy would lead to severe hypertension were it not accompanied by vasodilatation. The single greatest cardiovascular change in pregnancy is vasodilatation, resulting in a net decrease in systemic blood pressure during the midtrimester. The mechanism of vasodilatation is disputed but may depend on a variety of endothelial mechanisms including enhanced production of vasodilatory prostanoids, nitric oxide and activation of the endothelium-derived hyperpolarising factor channels (Kenny et al. 2002). Cardiac drugs that intercept or augment any of these mechanisms may have an effect on the vasculature of a pregnant woman. Perfusion of different organs is disproportionately enhanced in pregnancy and drugs that change blood pressure may have disproportionate effects on perfusion in different vascular beds. This may be of direct relevance to uterine and choriodecidual perfusion in the placental bed.

Increased Organ Perfusion

Three vascular beds show evidence of increased blood flow. The uterine perfusion increases tenfold increase by the time term is reached (Assali et al. 1960). The kidney also has a 50 % increase in blood flow while the skin shows evidence of increased perfusion (Davison and Noble 1981). These changes reflect the mechanism of renal adaptation to pregnancy, the process of thermoregulation necessitated by enhanced metabolism as well as the delivery of oxygen and nutrients to the fetus.

Protein Binding

Changes in Serum Protein Concentration

Serum albumin concentrations fall during pregnancy and drugs that bind to serum albumin are present in higher free concentrations. Some of these effects may not be solely related to changes in serum protein concentration but the presence of competitive endogenous inhibitors of drug binding. Albumin binds drugs in two main binding sites with warfarin, digoxin and furosemide being among those bound to subdomain IIa.

Changes in Drug Transporter Proteins

Transporter proteins are expressed on the apical and basal aspects of epithelial cells where they facilitate the movement of endogenous and exogenous substances from the blood into the cells and vice versa (Feghali and Mattison 2011). These proteins may be subject to induction and inhibition by exogenous drugs as well as genetic variation in expression. The placental transporter proteins also show variation in expression with increasing gestational age (Feghali and Mattison 2011).

Metabolic Rate and Metabolism

Cytochrome P450 is the most important system responsible for drug metabolism. While certain of the enzymes associated with this system show increased activity (CYP3A4 and CYP2D6), others have decreased levels of activity (CYP1A2). Hence, nifedipine metabolised by CYP3A4 will have lower trough levels than seen in non-pregnant women given the same dose. The enzyme system involving uridine 5′ -diphosphate glucuronosyltransferase (UGT) is also induced by pregnancy and may accelerate the metabolism of substrate drugs (Feghali and Mattison 2011).

Renal Excretion

Glomerular filtration and effective renal plasma flow increase by 60–80 % during pregnancy. Drugs excreted in the urine may be more rapidly cleared from the plasma. In particular atenolol and digoxin show increased clearance although the changes are not arithmetically predictable due to the confounding effects of glomerular filtration, tubular secretion and reabsorption of individual drugs.

The Effect of Co-morbidity Arising from Obstetric Disease

Various obstetric and medical disorders may give rise to changes in pregnancy physiology which may in turn affect the use of drugs needed in the treatment of cardiovascular disease. Hence, renal and liver failure may complicate pregnancies affected by pre-eclampsia and fatty liver of pregnancy. Obstetric haemorrhage can result in a coagulopathic state and renal failure. Cardiac disease may arise from pregnancy complications which included pre-eclampsia (both diastolic and systolic dysfunction) while peripartum cardiomyopathy causes impaired systolic function.

Teratogenesis and Fetal Adverse Effects

Teratogenesis arises during embryogenesis. The first 2 weeks after conception are not associated with the risk of teratogenesis possibly because the maternal use of drugs in the pre-implantation phase of pregnancy limits fetal exposure to the drug (Rakusan 2010).

The overall risk of major malformations is cited at 1–3 % of all births with 1 % of these abnormalities being attributable to drugs ingested during pregnancy. Drugs are commonly used during pregnancy but only a relatively small number of the available drugs are known teratogens.

TABLE I United States Food And Drug Administration classification of drug teratogenicity

Category	Definition
A	Adequate, well-controlled studies in pregnant women have not shown an increased risk of fetal abnormalities in any trimester of pregnancy.
B	Animal studies have revealed no evidence of harm to the fetus; however, there have not been any adequate and well-controlled studies performed in pregnant women.
C	Animal studies have shown an adverse effect; however, there have not been any adequate and well-controlled studies in pregnant women, or no animal studies have been conducted and there have not been any adequate and well-controlled studies in pregnant women.
D	Adequate, well-controlled or observational studies in pregnant women have demonstrated a risk to the fetus. However, the benefits of therapy may outweigh the potential risk. For example, the drug may be acceptable if needed in a life-threatening situation or serious disease for which safer drugs cannot be used or are ineffective.
X	Adequate, well-controlled or observational studies in animals or pregnant women have demonstrated positive evidence of fetal abnormalities or risks. The use of the product is contraindicated in women who are or may become pregnant.

The teratogenic effects of drugs are classified by the United States Food and Drug Administration into categories of risk based upon available evidence (see Table 1).

Two drugs used in the management of cardiovascular disease are known to be associated with teratogenic effects. Angiotensin converting enzyme inhibitors may lead to tubular dysgenesis and decreased skull ossification (Koren et al. 1998). This may result in prolonged neonatal renal failure. Angiotensin II receptor blockers and direct renin inhibitors should be considered to have the same risks as the ACE inhibitors. In general, ACE inhibitors are regarded as contraindicated during pregnancy. The evidence of malformation arising from the inadvertent use of these drugs in the first trimester is contradictory and prior exposure to ACE inhibitors is not usually regarded as an indication for termination of pregnancy (Rakusan 2010).

Warfarin is a clearly identified teratogen giving rise to nasal hypoplasia when used in the first trimester. It may also cause calcification of the fetal long-bone epiphysis (chondroplasia punctata) (Rakusan 2010). Warfarin will anticoagulate the fetal circulation and increase the risk of fetal haemorrhage. This can result in intrauterine death or the delivery of a neonate with cerebral haemorrhage.

There is evidence that antihypertensive drugs used in the first trimester are associated with a higher risk of fetal disease including Ebstein malformation, coarctation of the aorta, pulmonary valvular stenosis and atrial septal defects. Nevertheless, antihypertensive drugs are mostly classified as FDA category C agents (Caton et al. 2009). Beta-blockers are generally regarded as safe with the exception of atenolol which has been implicated in the development of intrauterine growth restriction.

Antiarrhythmic drugs have been variably classified by the FDA. Hence, sotalol (potassium blocking agent) is category B while amiodarone, in the same group of antiarrhythmic drugs is associated with fetal hypothyroidism and prematurity. Class IV anti-arrhythmic drugs such as calcium channel blockers are in FDA category C and generally regarded as safe (Rakusan 2010). The same applies to the Class II antiarrhythmic drugs – the beta blockers that also classify into Category C. The exception to this rule is atenolol. Class I anti-arrhythmic drugs (sodium channel blockers) are also classified into Category C. These include quinidine, procainamide and lidocaine (Rakusan 2010).

General Principles of Prescribing in Pregnancy

Only clearly-indicated drugs of proven efficacy and safety should be prescribed in pregnancy. Every effort should be made to avoid the use of drugs during the first trimester and where pregnant women have been exposed to known teratogens the risks of adverse outcome should be disclosed and considered by the physician and his/her client.

The efficacy of drugs used during pregnancy may be altered by pregnancy and attention should be paid to the adjustment of doses and the possible effects of drugs on the fetus once they have crossed the placenta.

References

Anderson GD. Pregnancy-induced changes in pharmacokinetics. Clin Pharmacokinet. 2005;44(10):989–1008.

Assali NS, Rauramo L, Peltonen T. Uterine and fetal blood flow and oxygen consumption in early human pregnancy. Am J Obstet Gynecol. 1960;79:86.

Caton AR, Bell EM, Druschel CM, et al. Antihypertensive medication use during pregnancy and the risk of cardiovascular malformations. Hypertension. 2009;54:63–70.

Davison JM, Noble MC. Serial changes in 24-hour creatinine clearance during normal menstrual cycles and the first trimester of pregnancy. Br J Obstet Gynaecol. 1981;88:10.

de Swiet M. The cardiovascular system. In: Hytten F, Chamberlain G, editors. Clinical physiology in obstetrics. Oxford: Blackwell Scientific Publications; 1980.

Feghali MN, Mattison DR. Clinical therapeutics in pregnancy. J Biomed Biotechnol. 2011:783528. doi:10.1155/2011/783528. Published online 2011 July 6.

Isoherranen N, Thummel KE. Drug metabolism and transport during pregnancy: how does drug disposition change during pregnancy and what are the mechanisms that cause such changes? Drug Metab Dispos. 2013;41:256–62.

Kenny LC, Baker PN, Kendall DA, Randall MD, Dunn WR. Mechanisms of endothelium-dependent vasodilator responses in human myometrial small arteries in normal pregnancy and pre-eclampsia. Clin Sci (Lond). 2002;103(1):67–73.

Koren G, Pastuszak A, Ito S. Drugs in pregnancy. N Engl J Med. 1998;338(16):1128–37.

Mabie WC, DiSessa TG, Crocker LG, et al. A longitudinal study of cardiac output in normal human pregnancy. Am J Obstet Gynecol. 1994;170:849.

Rakusan K. Drugs in pregnancy: implications for a cardiologist. Exp Clin Cardiol. 2010;15(4):e100–e103.

Sibai BM, Frangieh A. Maternal adaptation to pregnancy. Curr Opin Obstet Gynecol. 1995;7:420.

Management of Hypertension

Eckhart J. Buchmann

Epidemiology and Pathogenesis

High blood pressure affects about 10 % of pregnancies worldwide (Duley 2009), and is the second-most frequent cause of maternal death (Khan et al. 2006). The most serious form of pregnancy hypertension is pre-eclampsia, a progressive multisystem disorder only curable by delivery of the infant. Pre-eclampsia is found in about 2–8 % of pregnancies (Duley 2009), with 5–8 % of pre-eclamptic women in less-developed countries going on to eclamptic convulsions (World Health Organization 2011). Other complications of pre-eclampsia include intracerebral haemorrhage, pulmonary oedema, liver rupture, placental abruption, fetal growth restriction, and HELLP (haemolysis, elevated liver enzymes, low platelets) syndrome.

Factors associated with a high risk for developing pre-eclampsia include a previously affected pregnancy, family history of pre-eclampsia, thrombophilia, multiple pregnancy, and pre-existing chronic hypertension. Pre-eclampsia originates from abnormal placental development, possibly

E.J. Buchmann, MBBCh, FCOG (SA), MSc (Epidemiology), PhD
Department of Obstetrics and Gynaecology,
University of the Witwatersrand, 7 York Road, Parktown,
Johannesburg 2193, South Africa
e-mail: eckhart.buchmann@wits.ac.za

K. Sliwa, J. Anthony (eds.), *Cardiac Drugs in Pregnancy*,
Current Cardiovascular Therapy,
DOI 10.1007/978-1-4471-5472-3_2,
© Springer-Verlag London 2014

explained by immune factors, oxidative stress, placental enzyme (haemoxygase-1) abnormalities or chronic placental hypoxia (Powe et al. 2011). The essential defect is failure of placental cytotrophoblast cells to invade uterine spiral artery muscular walls early in pregnancy. Normally, invasion of the spiral artery walls provides the placenta with high-flow low-resistance feeder vessels that facilitate placental growth and function. Defective spiral artery invasion results in poor placental function, suboptimal fetal growth, and the maternal syndrome of pre-eclampsia. The mechanism of disease for the maternal syndrome appears to be the release of antiangiogenic factors (soluble FMS-like tyrosine kinase-1 and soluble endoglin) from the diseased placenta into the maternal circulation (Powe et al. 2011; Pennington et al. 2012). These factors bind maternal angiogenic factors (vascular endothelial growth factor, placental growth factor, transforming growth factor-beta), and inhibit the angiogenic factors' endothelial maintenance functions. The result is endothelial damage, vasospasm, capillary leakiness, and vessel wall platelet aggregation in multiple organ systems. This occurs most notably in the kidney, brain, liver, and uteroplacental circulation, leading to hypertension, proteinuria, oedema, and thrombocytopaenia, with the clinical complications as mentioned above. Overall, the pre-eclamptic woman's circulation becomes contracted, with reduced plasma volume and underperfusion of vital organs.

Definitions and Classification of Hypertensive Disorders of Pregnancy

Not all women with hypertension in pregnancy have pre-eclampsia. To plan clinical management, knowledwge of the spectrum of pregnancy hypertensive disorders and their classification is necessary. These disorders can be grouped into three categories: pre-eclampsia, gestational hypertension and pre-existing hypertension. The definitions and classification given below are based on those of the Society for Obstetric Medicine of Australia and New Zealand (SOMANZ), the

American College of Obstetricians and Gynecologists (ACOG), and the European Society of Cardiology (ESC) (SOMANZ 2008; American College of Obstetricians and Gynecologists 2002; The Task Force on the Management of Cardiovascular Diseases during Pregnancy of the European Society of Cardiology (ESC) 2011).

Definitions

Hypertension in pregnancy is defined as a systolic blood pressure (BP) $\geq$140 mmHg, and/or a diastolic BP $\geq$90 mmHg, confirmed by repeated findings of elevated BP over several hours. Severe hypertension is defined as a systolic BP $\geq$160 mmHg and/or a diastolic BP $\geq$110 mmHg. The BP should be recorded with the woman sitting or in a semi-lateral position with the inflatable cuff at the level of the heart, using Korotkoff 5 for diastolic BP. The gold standard recording method is a mercury sphygmomanometer. Automated BP measurement devices may be used, but should be calibrated regularly against a mercury sphygmomanometer to ensure reliable BP recordings.

Proteinuria in the context of hypertension in pregnancy is defined as urinary protein excretion $\geq$300 mg in 24 h, or a spot urine protein:creatinine ratio $\geq$30 mg/mmol, or, in the absence of laboratory services, persistent proteinuria $\geq$1+ (30 mg/dL) on urine reagent strips.

Classification

Pre-eclampsia is new-onset hypertension, with proteinuria or organ system dysfunction (Table 1), arising after 20 weeks of gestation. Severe pre-eclampsia is pre-eclampsia with BP $\geq$160/110 mmHg or organ system dysfunction (American College of Obstetricians and Gynecologists 2002). The term 'mild pre-eclampsia' is sometimes used to describe pre-eclampsia with BP <160/110 mmHg and no evidence of organ dysfunction (Koopmans et al. 2009).

TABLE I Definition of pre-eclampsia

Pre-eclampsia is new-onset hypertension (BP $\geq$140/90 mmHg) that arises after 20 weeks of gestation and is accompanied by at least one of the following (SOMANZ 2008):

Renal involvement

    Proteinuria

    Oliguria

    Serum creatinine $\geq$90 µmol/L

Haematological involvement

    Thrombocytopaenia

    Haemolysis

    Disseminated intravascular coagulation

Liver involvement

    Raised serum transaminases

    Severe epigastric or right upper quadrant pain

    Liver subcapsular haemorrhage or rupture

Neurological involvement

    Convulsions (eclampsia)

    Hyperreflexia with sustained clonus

    Visual disturbances

    Stroke

Cardiorespiratory involvement

    Pulmonary oedema

Uteroplacental involvement

    Fetal growth restriction

    Placental abruption

Gestational hypertension is new-onset hypertension arising after 20 weeks of gestation, with no evidence of proteinuria and no organ dysfunction. The ESC guidelines consider pre-eclampsia as a proteinuric or multisystem-involved subgroup of gestational hypertension (The Task Force on the Management of Cardiovascular Diseases during Pregnancy of the European Society of Cardiology (ESC) 2011).

Pre-existing (chronic) hypertension is hypertension known to have been present before the pregnancy, or new-onset hypertension detected before 20 weeks of gestation. This may be essential hypertension (no known cause) or hypertension secondary to cardiovascular, renal or endocrine disorders. When pre-existing hypertension is associated with increasing blood pressure or proteinuria after 20 weeks, this is termed superimposed pre-eclampsia.

It may be difficult to classify women who present themselves with new-onset hypertension only after 20 weeks of gestation. Follow up at 3 months after delivery is then necessary to confirm or exclude pre-existing hypertension.

General Principles in Managing Hypertension in Pregnancy

Initial Assessment

On presentation of a pregnant woman with hypertension, the two essential elements of management are to: (1) treat any presenting emergency; and (2) classify the hypertensive disorder to plan ongoing management (Fig. 1).

Emergencies associated with hypertension in pregnancy include eclampsia, severe hypertension, stroke, hypovolaemia from placental abruption or liver rupture, and acute pulmonary oedema. These conditions need to be managed appropriately according to local guidelines.

Most women presenting with hypertension in pregnancy have no or minimal symptoms, their hypertension having been detected on routine BP measurement at prenatal clinics. History-taking should include previous medical history; previous hypertension; known cardiovascular, endocrine or kidney disease; course and outcome of previous pregnancies; family history of hypertension, kidney disease or

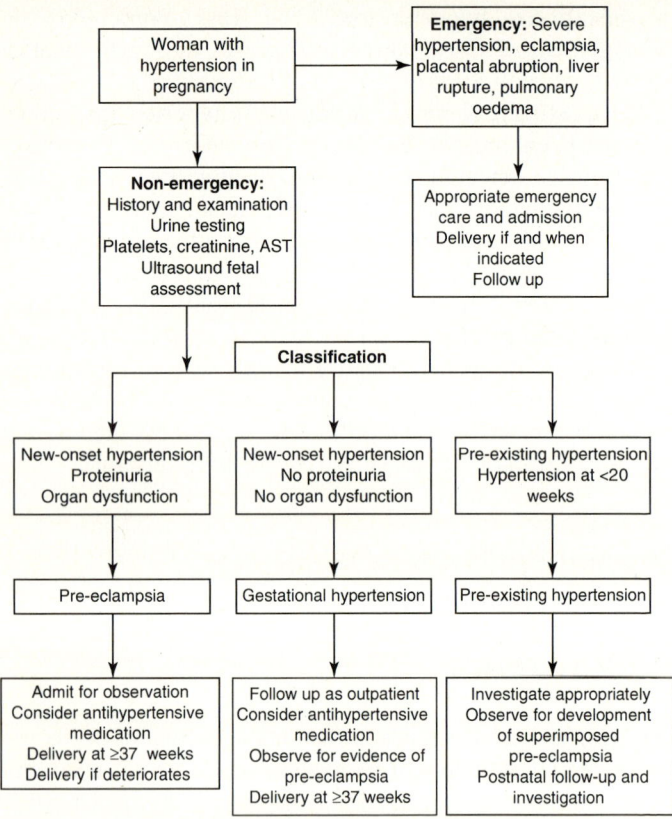

FIGURE I Initial assessment, classification and management of a woman presenting with hypertension in pregnancy. Women who cannot be classified because their blood pressure was not measured in the first half of pregnancy may be provisionally classified as pre-eclampsia or gestational hypertension, depending on the presence or absence of proteinuria and organ dysfunction. Such women should be followed up 3 months after delivery to determine if their hypertension is pre-existing or was pregnancy-related

thrombophilia; and symptoms associated with pre-eclampsia (Table 1). Physical examination, other than raised BP, may be entirely normal, but may detect clinical evidence of pre-existing hypertension. Oedema is a non-specific finding that is frequent in normal pregnancy, and, unless severe, should not be considered as evidence of pre-eclampsia (SOMANZ 2008; The Task Force on the Management of Cardiovascular Diseases during Pregnancy of the European Society of Cardiology (ESC) 2011).

Special investigations that help in classifying hypertensive orders include urine reagent strip testing for protein, or, preferably, spot urine protein:creatinine ratio. Blood investigations include haemoglobin level, platelet count, and serum creatinine and aspartate transaminase (AST). In settings with limited laboratory services, these blood tests may be omitted if the woman feels well and has a BP <160/110 mmHg, with no proteinuria and no clinical evidence of pre-eclampsia (Table 1). Assessment of uteroplacental involvement includes ultrasound fetal biometry, amniotic fluid volume assessment and umbilical artery Doppler indices. In low-resource settings, ultrasound fetal assessment can be omitted if there is no evidence of pre-eclampsia, and if uterine fundal growth is clinically assessed as normal.

The management principles of specific hypertensive disorders are discussed below, based on clinical experience and on evidence-based recommendations suggested by the World Health Organization (WHO) (Table 2).

Mild Pre-eclampsia

Women with mild pre-eclampsia are usually not at immediate risk for complications. However, remission will not occur while pregnancy continues, and deterioration is likely over subsequent days and weeks. Little is gained by continuation of pregnancy at term, and therefore elective delivery (usually labour induction) is recommended from 37 weeks of gestation (Koopmans et al. 2009). Women at less than 37 weeks are best observed in hospital, with regular monitoring of BP, twice-weekly blood tests for platelet count, creatinine and AST levels, and ultrasound fetal assessment every 2 weeks. Where home BP monitoring and urine testing is feasible,

TABLE 2 World Health Organization recommendations for management of pre-eclampsia and eclampsia, with GRADE assessment of evidence and strength of recommendation (World Health Organization 2011)

Recommendation	Quality of evidence	Strength of recommendation
In women with mild pre-eclampsia or mild gestational hypertension at term, induction of labour is recommended	Moderate	Weak
Strict bed rest is not recommended for improving pregnancy outcomes in women with hypertension (with or without proteinuria)	Low	Weak
Women with severe hypertension in pregnancy should receive treatment with antihypertensive drugs	Very low	Strong
The choice of antihypertensive for severe hypertension in pregnancy should be based primarily on the clinician's experience, considering also cost and local availability	Very low	Weak
In women with severe pre-eclampsia at term, early elective delivery is recommended	Low	Strong
In women with severe pre-eclampsia, a viable fetus and before 34 weeks of gestation, expectant management is recommended, provided that uncontrolled hypertension, worsening organ dysfunction and fetal distress are absent and can be monitored	Very low	Weak
In women with severe pre-eclampsia at 34–36 weeks of gestation, expectant management may be recommended, provided that uncontrolled hypertension, worsening organ dysfunction and fetal distress are absent and can be monitored	Very low	Weak

Table 2 (continued)

Recommendation	Quality of evidence	Strength of recommendation
Elective termination of pregnancy is recommended for women with severe pre-eclampsia at a gestational age where the fetus is not viable or unlikely to achieve viability within 1–2 weeks	Very low	Strong
Magnesium sulphate is recommended for prevention of eclampsia in women with severe pre-eclampsia in preference to other anticonvulsants	High	Strong
Magnesium sulphate is recommended for treatment of women with eclampsia in preference to other anticonvulsants	Moderate	Strong

GRADE quality of evidence and recommendation definitions (Guyatt et al. 2008):

Quality of evidence:

High: further research is very unlikely to change confidence in the estimate of effect

Moderate: further research is likely to have an important effect on confidence in the estimate of effect and may change the estimate

Low: further research is very likely to have an important impact on confidence in the estimate of effect and is likely to change the estimate

Very low: any estimate of effect is very uncertain

Recommendation:

Strong: desirable effects of an intervention clearly outweigh the undesirable effects, or clearly do not.

Weak: desirable and undesirable effects are closely balanced

women may be assessed twice weekly as outpatients. There is uncertainty about the value of antihypertensive drug treatment for mild pre-eclampsia (Abalos et al. 2007) (discussed below). There is no evidence to support bed rest in the management of pre-eclampsia (Meher et al. 2005).

Severe Pre-eclampsia

The first priority in caring for pregnant women with severe pre-eclampsia is maternal stabilization, in particular lowering the BP to <160/110 mmHg. This is achieved with intravenous or short-acting oral antihypertensive drugs, followed by maintenance therapy with oral agents (discussed below). Magnesium sulphate is frequently given during stabilization, to prevent eclamptic convulsions (discussed below). For severe pre-eclampsia, hospital admission is mandatory, with close observation of maternal and fetal condition at referral level by obstetricians experienced in managing severe pre-eclampsia (Society for Maternal-Fetal Medicine and Sibai 2011). Severe pre-eclampsia places the woman and fetus at immediate threat of complications, and deterioration requiring delivery can be expected within 1–2 weeks. Once a woman is classified as having severe pre-eclampsia, she retains that classification until she delivers. Successful lowering of an elevated BP does not convert the woman to a mild category.

Early elective delivery is advised for pregnancies at term (≥37 weeks). At <37 weeks, an expectant approach is appropriate in the absence of complications. However, from 34 to 36 weeks, the risks of continuing pregnancy may be greater than the risks of prematurity for the newborn, hence the threshold for delivery is lower than at <34 weeks. If there are complications or organ system deterioration (persistent symptoms and signs, worsening kidney or liver function, eclampsia, pulmonary oedema, or deteriorating fetal condition), emergency delivery, often by caesarean section, is indicated, irrespective of gestational age (Society for Maternal-Fetal Medicine and Sibai 2011). With expectant management at <34 weeks, intramuscular betamethasone is given for 24 h before delivery to accelerate fetal lung maturity (Roberts and Dalziel 2006). In women with severe pre-eclampsia with a non-viable fetus (20–22 weeks, up to 26 weeks in low-resource settings), elective termination of pregnancy is advised in the maternal interest.

HELLP Syndrome

Women with severe pre-eclampsia who have thrombocyto-paenia and a raised AST level, or who appear ill (nausea, vomiting, pallor) should be further tested for haemolysis (haptoglobin and serum lactate dehydrogenase levels, peripheral blood smear). Evidence of haemolysis suggests HELLP syndrome, a microangiopathic form of severe pre-eclampsia. In HELLP syndrome, delivery is indicated, irrespective of gestational age, as soon as maternal condition is stabilized (Society for Maternal-Fetal Medicine and Sibai 2011). However, the syndrome may continue to deteriorate in the first 2 days after delivery. A strong case has been made for intramuscular dexamethasone rescue treatment as specific treatment for HELLP syndrome (Martin 2013), despite findings of a Cochrane systematic review that suggested little beneficial effect (Woudstra et al. 2010).

Eclampsia

Eclamptic convulsions are generalized tonic-clonic seizures indistinguishable from epileptic convulsions. Other causes of convulsions should always be considered, especially if the seizures are atypical. Computerized tomography or magnetic resonance imaging scanning may be recommended to exclude other causes of convulsions, or to detect cerebral damage associated with eclampsia. Immediate care for eclampsia is left lateral positioning, and oxygen by mask. Intravenous magnesium sulphate is the treatment of choice to prevent further convulsions (discussed below). Full clinical, laboratory and ultrasound assessment for pre-eclampsia, and appropriate treatment of severe hypertension, are part of initial management of eclampsia. Pregnancy should not be allowed to continue (SOMANZ 2008), and delivery is indicated within about 12 h of the first convulsion, vaginally or by caesarean section, depending on obstetric considerations. Intensive care unit admission and/or artificial ventilation may be needed for women who do not regain consciousness rapidly after convulsions, or who have co-existent complications of severe pre-eclampsia.

Gestational Hypertension

Women with gestational hypertension have no abnormalities other than a raised BP. Some go on to develop pre-eclampsia. Weekly attendance as outpatients is recommended with BP measurement, urine testing for protein, and, if feasible, blood testing for platelet count, creatinine and AST. Four-weekly ultrasound fetal assessment may give some reassurance. As with mild pre-eclampsia, there is uncertainty about the place and value of antihypertensive drug treatment (Abalos et al. 2007). At ≥37 weeks of gestation, there is little benefit in continuing the pregnancy, and elective delivery is advised based on evidence from a large randomized trial (Koopmans et al. 2009).

Pre-existing Hypertension

Only limited investigations are possible in pregnancy for causes of pre-existing hypertension, and these should be based on clinical findings, focusing on renal, endocrine and cardiovascular causes. Where a secondary cause for hypertension is found, this may require expert medical management with appropriate specialists.

Women with uncomplicated essential hypertension are managed as for gestational hypertension, the most important concern being the development of superimposed pre-eclampsia. The physiological decrease in BP during the second trimester of pregnancy may allow antihypertensive drugs to be stopped, at least temporarily. However, in women with end-organ damage (heart, kidneys, optic fundi), antihypertensive treatment should be continued (Podymov and August 2011). For pre-existing hypertension, the recommended drugs are those used for mild hypertension in pregnancy (discussed below). Certain drugs may need to be discontinued and/or replaced. Angiotensin converting enzyme (ACE) inhibitors and angiotensin receptor blockers (ARBs) are contraindicated in pregnancy, having been implicated in fetal death and neonatal renal failure (Bullo et al. 2012). Selective beta-blockers such as atenolol may adversely affect fetal growth. Diuretics may interfere with physiological plasma volume expansion during pregnancy and should not be continued unless indicated for treatment of heart failure (SOMANZ 2008).

Pharmacological Management of Hypertension in Pregnancy

The choices for pharmacological treatment of hypertension in pregnancy are restricted to older, tried and tested drugs. Justifiable fears about adverse effects on the fetus have retarded research into the efficacy of newer drugs for hypertension in pregnancy, thus not allowing newer formulations into general use for these disorders.

Pharmacological management of hypertension in pregnancy is essentially the same irrespective of the classification of the hypertensive disorder, and is dictated by the level of the BP. It is recommended that individual clinicians or clinical units develop experience and expertise with a small range of the drugs that may be used, depending on cost and local availability (World Health Organization 2011). Information for discussion of the drugs below is sourced mainly from three authoritative reviews (Podymov and August 2011; Magee et al. 2011; SOMANZ 2008) and clinical experience.

Acute Blood Pressure Lowering for Severe Hypertension

A systolic BP ≥160 mmHg or diastolic BP ≥110 mmHg (severe hypertension) may overcome cerebral autoregulation and result in intracerebral haemorrhage or cerebral oedema. There is general agreement that severe hypertension needs urgent treatment. There is still some disagreement about the systolic BP cut-off level, with most guidelines favouring 160 mmHg, but at least one reputable guideline suggests 170 mmHg (SOMANZ 2008). The treatment goal is reduction in mean arterial pressure by <25 % over minutes to hours (Podymov and August 2011; Magee et al. 2011), with half-hourly monitoring of BP and heart rate. There are concerns that a rapid fall in BP might result in fetal distress, so a small preload of intravenous fluid, such as Ringer-Lactate 250 mL, may be given just before starting treatment (SOMANZ 2008). Fluid loading and plasma volume expansion are otherwise not recommended in managing pre-eclampsia, and excessive fluid loads may precipitate pulmonary oedema.

A Cochrane systematic review of randomized trials found little difference in effect between different drugs used for severe hypertension in pregnancy (Duley et al. 2006). Those most frequently compared were intravenous labetalol, oral nifedipine and intravenous hydralazine. The Cochrane reviewers recommended that choice of antihypertensive drugs should depend on local experience and familiarity with the different agents, but discouraged use of diazoxide, ketanserin, nimodipine and magnesium sulphate. A summary of drugs used in severe hypertension is given in Table 3.

Labetalol

Labetalol is a non-selective beta-blocker with alpha-1 receptor blocker activity. There have been reports of neonatal bradycardia, but these effects did not have clinical consequences (Magee et al. 2011). Labetalol should not be used in women with asthma or with congestive cardiac failure.

TABLE 3 Drugs used for acute blood pressure lowering in severe hypertension (BP ≥160/110 mmHg) in pregnancy, in descending order of preference (SOMANZ 2008; Podymov and August 2011; Magee et al. 2011)

Drug	Dose and route	Onset of action
Labetalol	20 mg IV over 2 min, repeat if necessary every 30 min with 20–80 mg, to a maximum of 300 mg/day. An infusion regimen may also be used	5 min
Nifedipine	5–10 mg capsules orally swallowed, repeat if necessary every 30 min, with 10 mg, to a maximum of 120 mg/day	10–20 min
Hydralazine	5 mg IV, repeat if necessary every 30 min with 5–10 mg, with a maximum dose of 20 mg	20 min
Diazoxide	30–50 mg IV every 5–15 min	3–5 min
Sodium nitroprusside[a]	0.25–5 µg/kg/min IV infusion, titrated to blood pressure response	Near-immediate

IV intravenous
[a]Sodium nitroprusside is a rarely used last-resort drug, with potential fetal toxicity, given in intensive care settings ideally after delivery of the infant

Nifedipine

Nifedipine is the only calcium channel blocker for which there is extensive experience in treating severe hypertension in pregnancy. Short-acting oral nifedipine 5 or 10 mg capsules are given orally to be swallowed. Sublingual administration may cause hypotension. Side-effects of oral nifedipine include headache and tachycardia. The capsules cannot be used if the woman is unable to swallow, and are best avoided in the presence of tachycardia (≥120/min), coronary artery disease or fixed cardiac output valvular disease. Theoretical fears of serious interactions with magnesium sulphate have not been realised in practice, and the simultaneous use of the two agents, for example in eclampsia accompanied by severe hypertension, is acceptable. Nicardipine is a calcium channel blocker that may be given intravenously to control severe hypertension in pregnancy (Nij Bijvank and Duvekot 2010).

Hydralazine

Hydralazine is a direct vasodilator of arteriolar smooth muscle. Intravenous use has been associated with maternal hypotension and fetal distress. Side effects include tachycardia, headache, and nausea. As with nifedipine, hydralazine is best avoided in the presence of tachycardia ($\geq$120/min) or fixed cardiac output valvular disease.

Other Drugs

Diazoxide is rarely used, and may cause a rapid drop in BP. Magnesium sulphate has little antihypertensive effect and should not be considered as an antihypertensive drug for pre-eclamptic women. Sodium nitroprusside is potentially valuable as a last resort treatment in an intensive care setting with intra-arterial BP monitoring. The main concern is fetal cyanide poisoning, and therefore, the drug should ideally only be used postpartum.

Treatment of Mild Hypertension, and Maintenance of Antihypertensive Effect

There is no certainty on the value of treating mild hypertension in pregnancy (140–159/90–109 mmHg). The WHO states explicitly in its guideline that no recommendation can be made, hence no statement appears in Table 2 (World Health Organization 2011). Importantly, antihypertensive treatment does not reduce progression to pre-eclampsia or severe pre-eclampsia. Theoretically, another benefit of treatment, besides BP reduction, could be vasodilatation with better organ system perfusion, and therefore prolongation of pregnancy. The harms of treatment may include reduction in uteroplacental blood flow, masking of progression of pre-eclampsia, and as yet

TABLE 4 Orally administered drugs frequently used for treatment of mild hypertension (BP 140–159/90–109 mmHg) in pregnancy, or for maintenance of antihypertensive effect after acute blood pressure lowering for severe hypertension, in descending order of preference (SOMANZ 2008; Podymov and August 2011; Magee et al. 2011)

Drug	FDA category	Dosage
Methyldopa	B	0.5–3.0 g/day in 2–4 divided doses. There is no evidence to support use of a loading dose.
Labetalol	C	200–1,200 mg/day in 2–3 divided doses
Nifedipine slow release	C	30–120 mg/day as a once-daily dose
Hydralazine	C	50–300 mg/day in 2–4 divided doses

United States of America Food and Drug Administration (FDA) drugs in pregnancy categories:

Category A: adequate and well-controlled studies have failed to show risk to the fetus in pregnancy.

Category B: animal studies have failed to show risk to the fetus but there are no adequate and well-controlled studies in humans.

Category C: animal studies have shown risk to the fetus, and there are no adequate and well-controlled studies in humans, but potential benefits may warrant use of the drug in pregnant women despite potential risks.

Category D: there is evidence of human fetal risk based on data from research or clinical experience, but potential benefits may warrant use of the drug in pregnant women despite potential risks.

Category X: studies in animals or humans have shown fetal abnormalities and/or there is evidence of human fetal risk based on research or clinical experience, and the risks involved in use of the drug in pregnant women clearly outweigh potential benefits.

unknown epigenetic effects on fetal programming that could increase risk of cardiovascular disease in later life (Magee et al. 2011). A frequent recommendation is that treatment should be considered in the higher range of 140–159/90–109 mmHg. For maintenance of antihypertensive effect in women who have been treated for severe hypertension, there is little doubt about the need for ongoing treatment. The drugs used are the same as those given for mild hypertension (Table 4).

Methyldopa

Methyldopa is a centrally acting alpha-2 adrenergic agonist prodrug that is converted to alpha-methylepinephrine, which replaces norepinephrine in adrenergic nerve terminals. Extensive experience and safety data exist for methyldopa used in pregnancy, including follow-up of children exposed during fetal life. Side-effects include depression, fatigue, dry mouth, and, rarely, haemolytic anaemia and hepatitis. Methyldopa is considered the first-line drug of choice by most authorities.

Beta-Blockers

The most commonly used beta-blocker is labetalol, backed up by extensive experience with the drug in pregnancy with a good safety record. There are still concerns about effects on uteroplacental flow and fetal growth. Side-effects include exercise intolerance, sleep disturbances and bronchoconstriction. The selective beta-blocker atenolol has been implicated in fetal growth restriction and is best avoided in pregnancy.

Calcium Channel Blockers

Slow-release nifedipine is the most favoured of the calcium channel blockers for treatment of mild hypertension. Other calcium channel blockers, for example amlodipine, have been used with safety and success, but have not matched the extensive experience gained with nifedipine used in pregnancy. Nifedipine is often used as a second-line drug ahead of labetalol. Side-effects include headache, tachycardia, palpitations and oedema.

Hydralazine

Oral hydralazine has a long history of use in pregnancy. It is now used mainly as a fourth-line agent in refractory cases of hypertension, owing to side-effects such as headache, nausea and palpitations, which may mimic symptoms of pre-eclampsia. Long-term use has rarely been associated with a polyneuropathy, and a lupus-like syndrome. Neonatal thrombocytopaenia and lupus have also been reported.

Other Drugs

Few other drugs are recommended. Prazosin and clonidine may occasionally be used. Thiazide diuretics are generally discouraged. ACE inhibitors and ARBs are implicated in cardiovascular teratogenesis if used in the first trimester, and in fetal death and neonatal renal failure if used later in pregnancy (Bullo et al. 2012), and are contraindicated in pregnancy.

Prevention and Treatment of Eclampsia

Magnesium sulphate is superior to other anticonvulsants (phenytoin and diazepam) for treatment and prevention of eclamptic convulsions. (The Collaborative Eclampsia Trial Group 1995). The exact mechanism of action of magnesium sulphate in eclamptic seizures in poorly understood, but could be related to cerebral vasodilatation, N-methyl-D-aspartate receptor antagonism, or calcium antagonism (James 2010).

Magnesium sulphate is given as an intravenous loading dose of 4 g in 200 mL saline, followed by an intravenous infusion at 1 g/h for up to 24 h after delivery, or for 24 h after the convulsion if the convulsion occurred postpartum. Where convulsions persist after magnesium loading, an additional dose of magnesium sulphate 2 g may be given intravenously, with clonazepam 1 mg over 5 min intravenously if necessary. In low-resource settings with limited monitoring capacity, intramuscular magnesium sulphate can be used with equivalent effect. A loading dose of 4 g IV is given as above, with 5 g intramuscularly in each buttock (total 14 g). This is followed by 4 hourly injections of 5 g into alternate buttocks for a total of 24 h after delivery or after the last postpartum convulsion.

Magnesium sulphate causes neuromuscular depression, and toxic levels may suppress respiration. While monitoring with magnesium levels is not necessary with the suggested dosage, hourly observation of respiratory rate and deep tendon reflexes is advised. Magnesium is only eliminated in the urine, so urine output must be monitored hourly using an indwelling urinary catheter, and magnesium sulphate infusion should be stopped with output <25 mL/h or <100 mL/4 h. If magnesium toxicity is suspected, airway management and ventilation may be required, with monitoring of serum magnesium levels. The antidote for magnesium toxicity is calcium gluconate 1 g given intravenously, repeated if necessary.

For prevention of eclampsia in women with severe pre-eclampsia, or with symptoms suggesting imminent convulsions (headache, visual disturbances, epigastric pain), magnesium sulphate has been shown to be effective in reducing the risk of convulsions, compared with placebo (Duley et al. 2010). Magnesium used for this indication is given in the same dosage as used for eclampsia, but need not be used for a full 24 h.

Antihypertensive Treatment After Delivery and During Breastfeeding

Pre-eclampsia and gestational hypertension do not remit immediately after delivery. It is therefore prudent to continue with antenatally prescribed antihypertensive medication during the early postpartum period. Medication may be adjusted if clinically indicated, for example if methyldopa is poorly tolerated. Pre-pregnancy medications that were discontinued during pregnancy may be restarted in women with pre-existing hypertension. Severe hypertension is treated as described above, although fetal considerations do not apply. Women may be discharged from hospital once the BP has settled at below 160/110 mmHg, with outpatient follow-up until the BP is normal. Hypertension that has not remitted by 3 months postpartum is likely to have been pre-existing and may require investigation.

There are theoretical and real concerns about antihypertensive drugs given during breastfeeding. The beta-blockers atenolol and acebutolol are concentrated in breastmilk and have been reported to cause neonatal hypotension, bradycardia and cyanosis (Beardmore et al. 2002). Other beta-blockers given to the mother, such as labetalol and propranolol, appear to be safe for the nursing infant. Diuretics reduce circulating blood volume and could reduce breastmilk volume, although there are insufficient data to support this contention. ACE inhibitor drugs are found in breastmilk in small quantities, but the American Academy of Paediatrics has passed captopril, enalapril and quinapril as safe during breastfeeding (American Academy of Pediatrics Committee on 2001). Caution is advised with prescribing these drugs in the 1st week or 2 after delivery, and for women who are breastfeeding preterm infants. ARBs should not be given to breastfeeding women, as there are insufficient data on safety. The other commonly used antihypertensive drugs (methyldopa, calcium channel blockers and hydralazine) appear to be safe (American Academy of Pediatrics Committee on 2001).

Future Therapeutic Possibilities for Pre-eclampsia

Recent advances in the understanding of the pathogenesis of pre-eclampsia have exposed new targets for therapeutic interventions to prevent or treat the syndrome. One such possibility is treatment with recombinant vascular endothelial growth factor, which has shown promise in a rat model (Young et al. 2010). A more realistic and exciting option is treatment with statins. The so-called pleiotropic effects of statins include positive effects on haemoxygenase-1, nitric oxide and angiogenic factors, as well as antioxidant activity.

These effects target critical pathways in the pathogenesis of pre-eclampsia (Lecarpentier et al. 2012). Statins have so far been contraindicated in pregnancy for fear of teratogenesis, but the first trial is now underway (the StAmP trial – Statins for the Amelioration of Pre-eclampsia) in the United Kingdom. In a double-blind placebo-controlled randomised trial, pravastatin is being given to women with early-onset pre-eclampsia. Obstetricians should eagerly await the results (Ahmed 2011).

References

Abalos E, Duley L, Steyn DW, Henderson-Smart DJ. Antihypertensive drug therapy for mild to moderate hypertension during pregnancy. Cochrane Database Syst Rev. 2007;1:CD002252.

Ahmed A. New insights into the etiology of preeclampsia: identification of key elusive factors for the vascular complications. Thromb Res. 2011;127 Suppl 3:S72–5.

American Academy of Pediatrics Committee on, Drugs. Transfer of drugs and other chemicals into human milk. Pediatrics. 2001;108:776–89.

American College of Obstetricians and Gynecologists. ACOG practice bulletin. Diagnosis and management of preeclampsia and eclampsia. Number 33, January 2002. Obstet Gynecol. 2002;99:159–67.

Beardmore KS, Morris JM, Gallery ED. Excretion of antihypertensive medication into human breast milk: a systematic review. Hypertens Pregnancy. 2002;21:85–95.

Bullo M, Tschumi S, Bucher BS, Bianchetti MG, Simonetti GD. Pregnancy outcome following exposure to angiotensin-converting enzyme inhibitors or angiotensin receptor antagonists: a systematic review. Hypertension. 2012;60:444–50.

Duley L. The global impact of pre-eclampsia and eclampsia. Semin Perinatol. 2009;33:130–7.

Duley L, Henderson-Smart DJ, Meher S. Drugs for treatment of very high blood pressure during pregnancy. Cochrane Database Syst Rev. 2006;3:CD001449.

Duley L, Gulmezoglu AM, Henderson-Smart DJ, Chou D. Magnesium sulphate and other anticonvulsants for women with pre-eclampsia. Cochrane Database Syst Rev. 2010;11:CD000025.

Guyatt GH, Oxman AD, Vist GE, Kunz R, Falck-Ytter Y, Alonso-Coello P, Schünemann HJ. GRADE: an emerging consensus on rating quality of evidence and strength of recommendations. BMJ. 2008;336: 1106–10.

James MF. Magnesium in obstetrics. Best Pract Res Clin Obstet Gynaecol. 2010;24:327–37.

Khan KS, Wojdyla D, Say L, Gulmezoglu AM, Van Look PF. World Health Organisation analysis of causes of maternal death: a systematic review. Lancet. 2006;367:1066–74.

Koopmans CM, Bijlenga D, Groen H, Vijgen SM, Aarnoudse JG, Bekedam DJ, van den Berg PP, de Boer K, Burggraaff JM, Bloemenkamp KW, Drogtrop AP, Franx A, de Groot CJ, Huisjes AJ, Kwee A, van Loon AJ, Lub A, Papatsonis DN, van der Post JA, Roumen FJ, Scheepers HC, Willekes C, Mol BW, van Pampus MG, HYPITAT Study Group. Induction of labour versus expectant monitoring for gestational hypertension or mild pre-eclampsia after 36 weeks' gestation (HYPITAT): a multicentre, open-label randomised controlled trial. Lancet. 2009;374:979–88.

Lecarpentier E, Morel O, Fournier T, Elefant E, Chavatte-Palmer P, Tsatsaris V. Statins and pregnancy: between supposed risks and theoretical benefits. Drugs. 2012;72:773–88.

Magee LA, Abalos E, von Dadelszen P, Sibai B, Easterling T, Walkinshaw S, CHIPS Study Group. How to manage hypertension in pregnancy effectively. Br J Clin Pharmacol. 2011;72:394–401.

Martin Jr JN. Milestones in the quest for best management of patients with HELLP syndrome (microangiopathic hemolytic anemia, hepatic dysfunction, thrombocytopenia). Int J Gynaecol Obstet. 2013;121: 202–7.

Meher S, Abalos E, Carroli G. Bed rest with or without hospitalisation for hypertension during pregnancy. Cochrane Database Syst Rev. 2005;4:CD003514.

Nij Bijvank SW, Duvekot JJ. Nicardipine for the treatment of severe hypertension in pregnancy: a review of the literature. Obstet Gynecol Surv. 2010;65:341–7.

Pennington KA, Schlitt JM, Jackson DL, Schulz LC, Schust DJ. Preeclampsia: multiple approaches for a multifactorial disease. Dis Model Mech. 2012;5:9–18.

Podymov T, August P. Antihypertensive drugs in pregnancy. Semin Nephrol. 2011;31:70–85.

Powe CE, Levine RJ, Karumanchi SA. Preeclampsia, a disease of the maternal endothelium: the role of antiangiogenic factors and implications for later cardiovascular disease. Circulation. 2011;123:2856–69.

Roberts D, Dalziel S. Antenatal corticosteroids for accelerating fetal lung maturation for women at risk of preterm birth. Cochrane Database Syst Rev. 2006;3:CD004454.

Society for Maternal-Fetal Medicine, Sibai B. Evaluation of management of severe pre-eclamsia before 34 weeks gestatation. Am J Obstet Gynecol. 2011;205:191–8.

SOMANZ Guidelines for the management of hypertensive disorders of pregnancy 2008. Society of Obstetric Medicine of Australia and New Zealand. 2008.

The Collaborative Eclampsia Trial Group. Which anticonvulsant for women with eclampsia? Evidence from the Collaborative Eclampsia Trial. Lancet. 1995;345:1455–63.

The Task Force on the Management of Cardiovascular Diseases during Pregnancy of the European Society of Cardiology (ESC). ESC guidelines on the management of cardiovascular diseases during pregnancy. Eur Heart J. 2011;32:3147–97.

World Health Organization. WHO recommendations for prevention and treatment of pre-eclampsia and eclampsia. Geneva: World Health Organization. 2011.

Woudstra DM, Chandra S, Hofmeyr GJ, Dowswell T. Corticosteroids for HELLP (hemolysis, elevated liver enzymes, low platelets) syndrome in pregnancy. Cochrane Database Syst Rev. 2010;9:CD008148.

Young BC, Levine RJ, Karumanchi SA. Pathogenesis of preeclampsia. Annu Rev Pathol. 2010;5:173–92.

Managing Heart Failure Pre- and Postpartum

Karen Sliwa and Kemilembe B. Tibazarwa

General Considerations

Introduction

Heart failure is the final common pathway of a large spectrum of diseases which can occur in pregnancy or in the immediate postpartum period. The spectrum of cardiovascular diseases (CVD) leading to heart failure in pregnancy and postpartum is changing and differs between regions of the world (Regitz-Zagrosek et al. 2011).

In the western world, the risk of having heart failure due to CVD has increased due to the increasing age of first pregnancy and increasing prevalence of cardiovascular risk factors. In addition, management of congenital heart disease has substantially improved, resulting in an increased number of women with congenital heart disease planning to have

K. Sliwa, MD, PhD, FESC, FACC (✉) • K.B. Tibazarwa, MD, MPH
Department of Medicine, Faculty of Health Sciences,
Hatter Institute for Cardiovascular Research in Africa,
Groote Schuur Hospital & University of Cape Town,
Observatory, Cape Town 7925, South Africa

Soweto Cardiovascular Research Unit,
Chris Hani Baragwanath Hospital,
University of the Witwatersrand, Johannesburg, South Africa
e-mail: sliwa-hahnlek@mdh-africa.org, http://www.hatter.uct.ac.za

K. Sliwa, J. Anthony (eds.), *Cardiac Drugs in Pregnancy*,   35
Current Cardiovascular Therapy,
DOI 10.1007/978-1-4471-5472-3_3,
© Springer-Verlag London 2014

children. However, some women with operated or not operated congenital heart disease are already in heart failure or develop heart failure while pregnant or in the postpartum period. In non-western countries, such as South Africa, rheumatic valvular disease dominates, comprising more than 50 % of all cardiac diseases in pregnancy presenting with heart failure (Nqayana et al. 2008; Soma-Pillay et al. 2008).

Cardiomyopathies often lead to cardiovascular complications in pregnancy. Women with previously diagnosed familial cardiomyopathy or peripartum cardiomyopathy have a serious risk of developing heart failure, leading to death in up to 30 % of cases. The aetiology of cardiomyopathies occurring in association with pregnancy is diverse – acquired as in peripartum cardiomyopathy (PPCM), genetic as in hypertrophic cardiomyopathy (HCM) or familial dilated cardiomyopathy (DCM).

This chapter will address counselling women who are at risk of developing heart failure or a known cardiomyopathy, general aspects of pharmacological and non-pharmacological management, as well as discuss novel data on the use of the dopamine D2-receptor antagonist, bromocriptine, in PPCM. The recommendations are based on the recently published European Society of Cardiology (ESC) Guidelines on the Management of Cardiovascular Disease During Pregnancy (Regitz-Zagrosek et al. 2011) and the ESC Guidelines for the Management of Grown-up Congenital Heart Disease (Baumgartner et al. 2010).

Management of Acute Heart Failure in Pregnancy

Heart failure in pregnant women with a pre-existing CVD can develop very rapidly and the guidelines for the management of acute heart failure include non-pharmacological and pharmacological intervention (Dickstein et al. 2008). Acute heart failure in pregnant women needs to be managed by a multi-disciplinary team of cardiologists, obstetricians, intensivists and anaesthesiologists. Any women presenting with shortness of breath in the post- partum period needs to be evaluated (Fig. 1, Table 1).

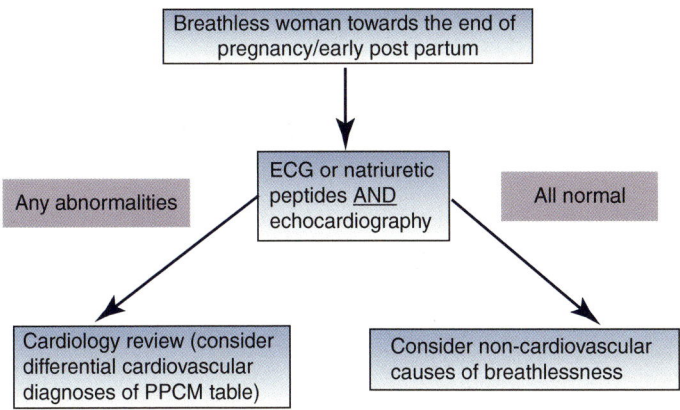

FIG. 1 Evaluation of a breathless woman towards the end of pregnancy/early postpartum

TABLE 1 Pre-conception evaluation and risk assessment in a women with heart failure

Pre-conception evaluation and risk management
Thorough history of cardiac symptoms and physical examination 12-lead ECG
Baseline exercise tolerance and functional class
Baseline echocardiogram
Assessment of ventricular function (right and left)
Assessment of pulmonary artery pressure
Presence and degree of valvular dysfunction
Assessment of stability of cardiac hemodynamic status over time
Effective contraception until pregnancy desired
Adjust medications to prevent adverse fetal events
Genetics referral for patients with heritable cardiac lesion

If a patient is hypotensive, or needing inotropes despite optimal medical therapy, she should be transferred to a facility where intra-aortic balloon pump counterpulsation, ventricular assist devices, and transplant consult teams are available.

Urgent delivery, irrespective of gestation, may need to be considered in women presenting or remaining in advanced heart failure with haemodynamic instability. As soon as the baby is delivered, and the patient is haemodynamically stable, standard therapy for heart failure can be applied.

Management of Chronic Heart Failure in Pregnancy

For treatment of chronic heart failure the pregnancy status of the patient is important. Patients can be peri- or postpartum. Women who present with heart failure during pregnancy require joint cardiac and obstetric care. Possible adverse effects on the fetus must be considered when prescribing drugs (Fig. 2; Tables 2 and 3).

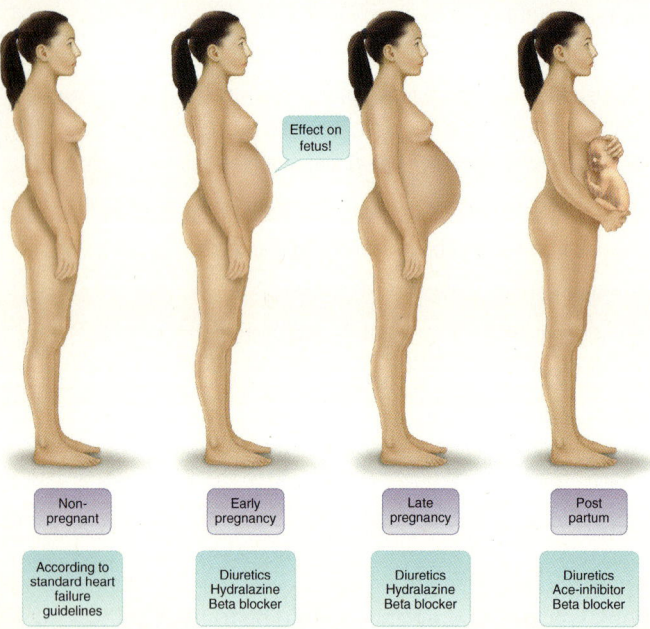

FIG. 2 Treatment of heart failure in women with peripartum cardiomyopathy or other cardiomyopathies according to stage of pregnancy

TABLE 2 Recommendations for the management of cardiomyopathies and heart failure in pregnancy

Recommendations	Level of evidence
CLASS I	
Anticoagulation is recommended in patients with intracardiac thrombus detected by imaging or with evidence of systemic embolism.	A
Women with HF during pregnancy should be treated according to current guidelines for non-pregnant patients, respecting contraindications for some drugs in pregnancy	B
Women with DCM should be informed about the risk of deterioration of the condition during gestation and peripartum.	C
In patients with a past history or family history of sudden death close surveillance with prompt investigation is recommended if symptoms of palpitations or presyncope are reported	C
Therapeutic anticoagulation with LMWH or vitamin K antagonists according to stage of pregnancy is recommended for patients with atrial fibrillation.	C
CLASS IIa	
Delivery should be performed with β-blocker protection in women with HCM.	C
β-blockers should be considered in all patients with HCM and more than mild LVOTO or maximal wall thickness >15 mm to prevent sudden pulmonary congestion	C
In HCM, cardioversion should be considered for persistent atrial fibrillation.	C

(continued)

TABLE 3 (continued)

Recommendations	Level of evidence
CLASS IIb	
Due to high metabolic demands of lactation and breastfeeding, preventing lactation may be considered in PPCM.	C
CLASS III	
Subsequent pregnancy is not recommended if LVEF does not normalize in women with PPCM.	C

Adapted from Regitz-Zagrosek et al. (2011)

DCM dilated cardiomyopathy, *HCM* hypertrophic cardiomyopathy, *HF* heart failure, *LMWH* low molecular weight heparin, *LVEF* left ventricular ejection fraction, *LVOTO* left ventricular outflow tract obstruction, *PPCM* peripartum cardiomyopathy

Level of evidence A: Data derived from multiple randomized clinical studies or meta-analysis

Level of evidence B: Data derived from single randomized clinical trial or large non-randomized studies

Level of evidence C: Consensus of opinion of experts and/or small studies, retrospective studies or registries

TABLE 3 Medical management of chronic heart failure in pregnancy according to *U.S. Food and Drug Administration (FDA) class*

Medical management of chronic heart failure in pregnancy		
Drug/class	**Purpose**	**Comments**
Diuretics		
Furosemide	Generally reserved for treatment of pulmonary edema	Can result in uteroplacental hypoperfusion
	Use of lowest possible dose	FDA class C[a]
Digoxin	Not considered first-line therapy for heart failure in non-pregnant patients	Generally considered safe
		Useful in treatment of persistent symptoms, despite standard therapy
	No improvement in mortality	FDA class C

Table 3 (continued)

Medical management of chronic heart failure in pregnancy		
Drug/class	**Purpose**	**Comments**
Vasodilators		
Hydralazine	Commonly used oral antihypertensive agent in pregnancy	Demonstrated efficacy in hypertension Risk of hypotension
	Can be substituted for ACE inhibitor during pregnancy	Avoid large or precipitous decreases in blood pressure FDA class C
Aldosterone antagonists		
Spironolactone, epleronone	Prolong survival in selected heart failure patients	Not routinely used in pregnancy No data to support safety in pregnancy FDA class D
Warfarin	Risk/benefit ratio needs to be discussed with the patient for treatment and prophylactic anticoagulation in severe left ventricular dysfunction	First trimester teratogenesis Dosing is complicated in pregnancy FDA class X (contraindicated)

ACE angiotensin converting enzyme, *ARB* angiotensin receptor blocker, *IUGR* intrauterine growth retardation, *SVR* systemic vascular resistance

[a]U.S. Food and Drug Administration (FDA) class: A (controlled studies show no risk), B (no evidence of human risk in controlled studies), C (risk cannot be ruled out), D (positive evidence of risk), X (contraindicated in pregnancy)

Heart failure should be treated according to guidelines on acute and chronic heart failure (Gheorghiade et al. 2010). The principal objectives in the management of heart failure are to make patients feel better, reduce hospitalisations (new and recurrent) and to prolong survival. Drugs such as diuretics and digoxin improve symptoms. Beta-blockers, ACE-inhibitors and aldosterone antagonists improve survival. It is now recognized that preventing HF hospitalisation is important for patients and healthcare systems.

Data on the use of medications in pregnancy are limited as pharmaceutical studies often exclude pregnant women due to fear of litigation if fetal effects occur. Evidence is therefore limited and for most medication only a 'class C' (Consensus of opinion of experts and/or small studies, retrospective studies or registries) (Regitz-Zagrosek et al. 2011) is available. Levels of evidence on the recommendations for the management of cardiomyopathies and heart failure in pregnancy is summarized in Tables 2 and 3. A number of drugs commonly used in the management of chronic heart failure are not recommended during pregnancy.

Angiotensin Converting Enzyme (ACE) inhibitors, Angiotensin Receptor Blockers (ARBs), and renin inhibitors are contraindicated because of fetotoxicity (Cooper et al. 2006; Bullo et al. 2012).

A recent systemic review by Bullo et al. in Hypertension (Bullo et al. 2012) reported on the use of ACE-inhibitors and ARBs from a total of 72 reports. Thirty-seven articles on 118 well-documented cases described the prenatal exposure to ACE-inhibitors and 35 articles on 68 cases described the use of ARBs. Overall, 52 % of the newborns exposed to ACE-inhibitors and 13 % of the newborns exposed to ARBs did not exhibit any complications ($p < 0.0001$). Neonatal complications were more frequent following exposure to ARBs and included renal failure, oligohydramnions, death, arterial hypertension, intrauterine growth retardation, respiratory distress syndrome, pulmonary hypoplasia, limb defects and persistent patent ductus arteriosus. Fetal adverse effects by both drugs had relevant neonatal and long-term complications. The outcome was poorer following exposure to ARBs versus ACE-inhibitors. The authors rightly concluded that relevant complications are regularly described, indicating that awareness of the deleterious effects of prenatal exposure to drugs inhibiting the renin-angiotensin system should be improved.

For symptomatic relief, and to reduce afterload, hydralazine and nitrates can be used instead of ACE inhibitors/ARBs for afterload reduction. Diuretics should only be used if pulmonary congestion is present since they may decrease blood flow to the placenta. Furosemide and hydrochlorothiazide are most frequently used.

For symptomatic relief, managing tachycardia and improving long-term outcome, beta-blockers can be considered, carefully weighing up the benefit for the mother versus the possible impaired outcome for the fetus and newborn baby. Data on beta-blocker use in pregnancy are limited and conflicting. However, a recently published survey from a Danish birth cohort (Meidahl Petersen et al. 2012), comprising all births in Denmark between 1995 and 2008, explored the effect of beta-blockers on pregnancy outcomes. The authors identified 2,459 pregnancies exposed to beta-blockers. Interestingly, Danish pharmacies are required by law to register all redeemed prescriptions and, therefore, this study included data on exposure to beta-blockers based on information on prescriptions paid for and not only prescribed by the physician. The authors defined being born small for gestational age as having a birth weight below the 10th percentile for the corresponding gestational week. Preterm birth was defined as born before the 37th gestational week. Beta-blocker exposure during pregnancy was found to be associated with increased risk of small for gestational age (SGA) fetuses (adjusted OR 1.97, 95 % CI 1.75–2.23), preterm birth (adjusted OR 2.26, 95 % ci 2.03–2.52) and an increased perinatal mortality (adjusted OR 1.89, 95 % CI 1.25–2.84). The authors found similar risks irrespective of type of beta-blocker used. However, the study has a major limitation in the way that the authors could not adjust for the treatment indication and severity of the maternal disease, nor were they able to rule out confounding factors. Maternal disease could also possibly explain the findings.

Newborns of mothers who needed to be on beta-blockers while pregnant should be supervised for 24–48 h after delivery to exclude hypoglycaemia, bradycardia, and respiratory depression.

Another medication that has been shown to improve long-term survival in patients with heart failure, aldosterone antagonists, should be avoided (Mirshahi et al. 2002). Animal studies suggest that the blockade of mineralocorticoid hormone provokes teratogenesis in rat embryos. Spironolactone can also be associated with antiandrogenic effects in the first trimester. Data for eplerenone are lacking.

Digoxin can be used safely in pregnancy and can be considered to reduce heart rate. In acute heart failure dopamine and levosimendan can be used if inotropic drugs are needed.

Care should be taken with anticoagulation therapy in the immediate phase after delivery but, once the bleeding has stopped, it should be considered in patients with a very low contractility of the heart and, therefore, a very low ejection fraction (<30 %) because peripheral embolism, including cerebral embolism and ventricular thrombi, are frequent in patients with severely impaired systolic function. This is in part due to increased procoagulant activity in the peripartum phase (Brenner 2004).

Anticoagulation is clearly recommended in patients with documented intracardiac thrombus detected by imaging or evidence of systemic embolism (Dickstein et al. 2008), as well as in patients with paroxysmal or persistent atrial fibrillation. Low molecular weight heparin (LMWH) or vitamin K antagonists are recommended according to the stage of pregnancy to prevent stroke (see chapter "Anticoagulation in Pregnancy" by Prof. Vera Regitz-Zagrosek). When LMWH is used, anti-Xa levels should be monitored.

Breastfeeding

Some ACE inhibitors (benazepril, captopril, enalapril) have been sufficiently tested in breastfeeding women and use by the mother is safe for the baby (Regitz-Zagrosek et al. 2011; Beardmore et al. 2002). Weight monitoring of the child during the first 4 weeks is essential as an indicator of kidney dysfunction. A recent small prospective randomized pilot study supports the hypothesis that the addition of bromocriptine, which terminates lactation via inhibition of prolactin, in addition to standard heart failure therapy, has beneficial effects on ventricular function and clinical outcome in women with acute severe PPCM (Sliwa et al. 2010a). In addition, due to high metabolic demands of lactation and breast-feeding, preventing lactation may be considered.

Pre-conceptual Counselling for Women with Structural Heart Disease Receiving Medications

Women with any form of cardiomyopathy or heart failure should be informed about the risk of deterioration of the condition during gestation and peripartum (see below). They should be counselled based on individual risk stratification. Any pregnancy in patients with poor systolic function, such as a left ventricular systolic function (LVEF) <40 %, is a predictor of high risk and close monitoring in a tertiary centre should be advised. If LVEF is <20 %, maternal mortality is very high and termination of the pregnancy should be considered (Regitz-Zagrosek et al. 2011; Sliwa et al. 2010b). Women with mildly impaired systolic function wishing to fall pregnant and accepting the increased risk of maternal and fetal morbidity and mortality need to receive advice on medication that needs to be replaced (such as aldosterone antagonists, ACE-inhibitors and warfarin) due to documented teratogenic effects, prior to falling pregnant. They need to be referred and managed by a multi-disciplinary team of cardiologists, obstetricians and intensivists and carefully monitored throughout the pregnancy.

Pharmacological Management of Specific Cardiomyopathies in Pregnancy

Dilated Cardiomyopathy

Dilated cardiomyopathy (DCM) is defined by the presence of a dilated left ventricle, impaired systolic function and, often, typical symptoms of heart failure. The condition can be of unknown etiology or have a familial predisposition due to genetic changes. Differentiation from PPCM is often difficult and can sometimes only be achieved retrospectively. If not known before conception, the condition is most often unmasked during the first or second trimester when the hae-modynamic load is increased. A family history of DCM speaks in favour of the DCM diagnosis and against PPCM. Pregnancy outcome of women with a classical DCM in preg-nancy describe marked deterioration during pregnancy and a poor outcome (Grewal et al. 2009). A pregnancy in patients with a DCMO with poor systolic function, such as a left ven-tricular systolic function (LVEF) <40 %, is considered to be a predictor of high risk. If LVEF is <20 %, maternal mortality is very high and termination of the pregnancy should be con-sidered (Regitz-Zagrosek et al. 2011; Sliwa et al. 2010b).

Secondary cardiomyopathies such as infiltrative or toxic cardiomyopathies, arrhythmogenic right ventricular cardio-myopathy and other rare forms can also develop symptoms in pregnancy. At present data on continued use of beta-blocker therapy in patients with previously known DCM is scarce. Data from the ongoing ROPAC study by the European Cardiac Society via the Euro*Obs*-program (www.escardio.org) (Roos-Hesselink et al. 2013) will hopefully provide data on maternal and fetal outcome of women receiving beta-blocker therapy throughout their pregnancy.

Peripartum Cardiomyopathy

Peripartum cardiomyopathy (PPCM) is a life-threatening heart disease developing towards the end of pregnancy or in the months following delivery, in previously healthy women (Sliwa et al. 2010b). It is a diagnosis of exclusion when no other cause of heart failure is found. The LV may not be dilated, but the EF is nearly always reduced below 45 %. PPCM is the major cause of pregnancy-induced heart failure and is associated with high morbidity and mortality.

The true incidence of PPCM is unknown as clinical presen-tation varies. Current estimates range from 1:299 (Haiti),

1:1,000 (South Africa) to 1:3,186 (USA) pregnancies (Blauwet et al. 2013). No data exists on the frequency of the disease in Europe. Pathophysiology still remains unclear, with multiple factors likely to contribute to and to drive progression. Predisposing factors seem to be multiparity, family history, ethnicity, twin pregnancy and either advanced age of mothers or teenage pregnancy. Nevertheless, decisive advances have been achieved in understanding some underlying molecular cascades deregulated in PPCM (Sliwa et al. 2006a; Hilfiker-Kleiner et al. 2007a). The aetiology of PPCM is uncertain but inflammation and autoimmune processes may play a role (Sliwa et al. 2006b). Novel data on circulating microparticles released from cellular membranes during cell activity may be a diagnositic marker of disease (Walenta et al. 2012). PPCM is suspected to be the consequence of an unbalanced oxidative stress leading to proteolytic cleavage of the lactating hormone, prolactin, into a potent angiostatic factor and into pro-apoptotic fragments (Hilfiker-Kleiner et al. 2007a). Prolactin (PRL) can have opposing effects on angiogenesis, depending on proteolytic processing of the potentially pro-angiogenic full-length 23-kDa PRL into the antiangiogenic 16-kDa PRL. The role of 16-kDa PRL and the inhibition by the dopamine D2-receptor antagonist bromocriptine in animal models and human studies have recently been reviewed by Hilfiker-Kleiner et al. (2012).

Symptoms and signs are often typical for heart failure but, due to the special physiological situation of pregnancy and post-partum, a broad spectrum of symptoms is reported in PPCM patients. PPCM should be suspected in all women with a delayed return to the pre-pregnancy state. Frequently patients present with acute heart failure. Complex ventricular arrhythmias and sudden cardiac arrest are also described.

Recent case reports have indicated that the addition of bromocriptine to standard heart failure therapy may be beneficial in patients with acute onset PPCM (Hilfiker-Kleiner et al. 2007b). A proof-of-concept pilot study of PPCM patients with severely reduced LVEF, diagnosed within 1 month of delivery, showed a marked improvement in systolic function and reduced mortality in patients treated with bromocriptine

2.5 mg twice daily for 2 weeks, followed by 2.5 mg daily for 4 weeks, compared with patients receiving standard care with ACE-inhibitors and beta-blockers only. A larger randomized study is currently underway in order to confirm the previously reported beneficial effects of bromocriptine during the acute phase of PPCM and to assess whether these effects are enhanced by chronic bromocriptine therapy. PPCM patients are particularly vulnerable to thrombotic and thromboembolic complications due to pregnancy-induced hypercoagulability which begins during pregnancy, is heightened during labor and delivery, and persists up to several months postpartum. These patients not only have an increased risk of deep vein thrombosis and pulmonary embolism, they also have an increased risk for developing intracardiac thrombus, even if their systolic function is only moderately decreased (Sliwa et al. 2006b). Anticoagulation is not recommended for all PPCM patients but should be considered in patients with an LVEF <35 %. Case-reports associate bromocriptine in postpartum women with an increased risk for thrombotic events such as myocardial infarction (Hopp et al. 1996), which resulted in the drug being advocated as an agent to suppress/stop lactation in the United States. However, it is widely used in many Western European countries, Africa and Asia for this purpose and other indications, such as the treatment of Parkinson's disease. Recent studies suggest beneficial effect of bromocriptine being used in the therapy of adult patients with diabetes mellitus type 2 to diminish fasting glucose, improve glucose tolerance and being associated with reduction in cardiovascular morbidity (Gaziano et al. 2010). We feel that women with PPCM in general and, in particular, poor systolic function, should be considered for anticoagulation if INR monitoring can be offered, even if they are not receiving bromocriptine.

Hypertrophic Cardiomyopathy

Hypertrophic cardiomyopathy (HCM) is a common genetic disorder. The disease is frequently diagnosed for the first time in pregnancy by echocardiography. The most common substrates for complications are diastolic dysfunction due to the hypertrophied non-compliant myocardium, severe left ventricular outflow tract obstruction (LVOTO) and arrhythmias. Patients can present with symptoms that are typical for heart failure, with pulmonary congestion due to the increased end-diastolic pressure or syncope during physical activity. Echocardiography is the diagnostic tool of choice.

Women with HCM usually tolerate pregnancy well (Autore et al. 2002). Patients with a high risk clinical profile before pregnancy, i.e. having had a history of syncope or symptoms of heart failure, are at higher risk and need specialized obstetric care (Regitz-Zagrosek et al. 2011). Low risk cases may have a spontaneous labour and vaginal delivery.

Pharmacological management depends on symptoms and signs. Beta-blockers should be considered in patients with more than mild LVOTO and/or maximal wall thickness of >15 mm to prevent sudden pulmonary congestion during exertion or emotional stress (Spirito and Autore 2006). Beta-blockers should be used for rate control in AF and to suppress ventricular arrhythmias. Verapamil can be used as a second choice when beta-blockers are not tolerated but could cause AV block in the fetus. Cardioversion should be considered for persistent arrhythmia. Therapeutic anticoagulation with LMWH or vitamin K antagonists, according to stage of pregnancy, is recommended for those with paroxysmal or persistent AF. Patients with a past history or family history of sudden death need close surveillance with prompt investigation if symptoms of palpitations or pre-syncope are reported (Regitz-Zagrosek et al. 2011).

References

Autore C, Conte MR, Piccininno M, Bernabo P, Bonfiglio G, Bruzzi P, Spirito P. Risk associated with pregnancy in hypertrophic cardiomyopathy. J Am Coll Cardiol. 2002;40:1864–9.

Baumgartner H, Bonhoeffer P, De Groot NM, de Haan F, Deanfield JE, Galie N, Gatzoulis MA, Gohlke-Baerwolf C, Kaemmerer H, Kilner P, Meijboom F, Mulder BJ, Oechslin E, Oliver JM, Serraf A, Szatmari A, Thaulow E, Vouhe PR, Walma E, Task Force on the Management of

Grown-up Congenital Heart Disease of the European Society of, C., Association for European Paediatric, C. & Guidelines, E. S. C. C. f. P. ESC Guidelines for the management of grown-up congenital heart disease (new version 2010). Eur Heart J. 2010;31:2915–57.

Beardmore KS, Morris JM, Gallery ED. Excretion of antihypertensive medication into human breast milk: a systematic review. Hypertens Pregnancy. 2002;21:85–95.

Blauwet LA, Libhaber E, Forster O, Tibazarwa K, Mebazaa A, Hilfiker-Kleiner D, Sliwa K. Predictors of outcome in 176 South African patients with peripartum cardiomyopathy. Heart. 2013;99:308–13.

Brenner B. Haemostatic changes in pregnancy. Thromb Res. 2004;114:409–14.

Bullo M, Tschumi S, Bucher BS, Bianchetti MG, Simonetti GD. Pregnancy outcome following exposure to angiotensin-converting enzyme inhibitors or angiotensin receptor antagonists: a systematic review. Hypertension. 2012;60:444–50.

Cooper WO, Hernandez-Diaz S, Arbogast PG, Dudley JA, Dyer S, Gideon PS, Hall K, Ray WA. Major congenital malformations after first-trimester exposure to ACE inhibitors. N Engl J Med. 2006;354:2443–51.

Dickstein K, Cohen-Solal A, Filippatos G, McMurray JJ, Ponikowski P, Poole-Wilson PA, Stromberg A, van Veldhuisen DJ, Atar D, Hoes AW, Keren A, Mebazaa A, Nieminen M, Priori SG, Swedberg K, Vahanian A, Camm J, De Caterina R, Dean V, Dickstein K, Filippatos G, Funck-Brentano C, Hellemans I, Kristensen SD, McGregor K, Sechtem U, Silber S, Tendera M, Widimsky P, Zamorano JL, Tendera M, Auricchio A, Bax J, Bohm M, Corra U, della Bella P, Elliott PM, Follath F, Gheorghiade M, Hasin Y, Hernborg A, Jaarsma T, Komajda M, Kornowski R, Piepoli M, Prendergast B, Tavazzi L, Vachiery JL, Verheugt FW, Zamorano JL, Zannad F. ESC guidelines for the diagnosis and treatment of acute and chronic heart failure 2008: the Task Force for the diagnosis and treatment of acute and chronic heart failure 2008 of the European Society of Cardiology. Developed in collaboration with the Heart Failure Association of the ESC (HFA) and endorsed by the European Society of Intensive Care Medicine (ESICM). Eur J Heart Fail. 2008;10:933–89.

Gaziano JM, Cincotta AH, O'Connor CM, Ezrokhi M, Rutty D, Ma ZJ, Scranton RE. Randomized clinical trial of quick-release bromocriptine among patients with type 2 diabetes on overall safety and cardiovascular outcomes. Diabetes Care. 2010;33:1503–8.

Gheorghiade M, Follath F, Ponikowski P, Barsuk JH, Blair JE, Cleland JG, Dickstein K, Drazner MH, Fonarow GC, Jaarsma T, Jondeau G, Sendon JL, Mebazaa A, Metra M, Nieminen M, Pang PS, Seferovic P, Stevenson LW, van Veldhuisen DJ, Zannad F, Anker SD, Rhodes A, McMurray JJ, Filippatos G. Assessing and grading congestion in acute heart failure: a scientific statement from the acute heart failure committee of the heart failure association of the European Society of Cardiology and endorsed by the European Society of Intensive Care Medicine. Eur J Heart Fail. 2010;12:423–33.

Grewal J, Siu SC, Ross HJ, Mason J, Balint OH, Sermer M, Colman JM, Silversides CK. Pregnancy outcomes in women with dilated cardio-myopathy. J Am Coll Cardiol. 2009;55:45–52.

Hilfiker-Kleiner D, Kaminski K, Podewski E, Bonda T, Schaefer A, Sliwa K, Forster O, Quint A, Landmesser U, Doerries C, Luchtefeld M, Poli V, Schneider MD, Balligand JL, Desjardins F, Ansari A, Struman I, Nguyen NQ, Zschemisch NH, Klein G, Heusch G, Schulz R, Hilfiker A, Drexler H. A cathepsin D-cleaved 16 kDa form of prolactin medi-ates postpartum cardiomyopathy. Cell. 2007a;128:589–600.

Hilfiker-Kleiner D, Meyer GP, Schieffer E, Goldmann B, Podewski E, Struman I, Fischer P, Drexler H. Recovery from postpartum cardio-myopathy in 2 patients by blocking prolactin release with bromocrip-tine. J Am Coll Cardiol. 2007b;50:2354–5.

Hilfiker-Kleiner D, Struman I, Hoch M, Podewski E, Sliwa K. 16-kDa prolactin and bromocriptine in postpartum cardiomyopathy. Curr Heart Fail Rep. 2012;9:174–82.

Hopp L, Haider B, Iffy L. Myocardial infarction postpartum in patients taking bromocriptine for the prevention of breast engorgement. Int J Cardiol. 1996;57:227–32.

Meidahl Petersen K, Jiminez-Soilem E, Traerup Andersen J, Petersen M, Brodbaek K, Torp-Pedersen C, Poulsen H. Beta-blocker treatment during pregnancy and adverse pregnancy outcomes: a nation-wide population-based cohort study. BMJ Open. 2012;2(4):pii: e001185. doi:10.1136/bmjopen-2012-001185.

Mirshahi M, Ayani E, Nicolas C, Golestaneh N, Ferrari P, Valamanesh F, Agarwal MK. The blockade of mineralocorticoid hormone signaling provokes dramatic teratogenesis in cultured rat embryos. Int J Toxicol. 2002;21:191–9.

Nqayana T, Moodley J, Naidoo DP. Cardiac disease in pregnancy. Cardiovasc J Afr. 2008;19:145–51.

Regitz-Zagrosek V, Blomstrom Lundqvist C, Borghi C, Cifkova R, Ferreira R, Foidart JM, Gibbs JS, Gohlke-Baerwolf C, Gorenek B, Iung B, Kirby M, Maas AH, Morais J, Nihoyannopoulos P, Pieper PG, Presbitero P, Roos-Hesselink JW, Schaufelberger M, Seeland U, Torracca L, Bax J, Auricchio A, Baumgartner H, Ceconi C, Dean V, Deaton C, Fagard R, Funck-Brentano C, Hasdai D, Hoes A, Knuuti J, Kolh P, McDonagh T, Moulin C, Poldermans D, Popescu BA, Reiner Z, Sechtem U, Sirnes PA, Torbicki A, Vahanian A, Windecker S, Aguiar C, Al-Attar N, Garcia AA, Antoniou A, Coman I, Elkayam U, Gomez-Sanchez MA, Gotcheva N, Hilfiker-Kleiner D, Kiss RG, Kitsiou A, Konings KT, Lip GY, Manolis A, Mebaaza A, Mintale I, Morice MC, Mulder BJ, Pasquet A, Price S, Priori SG, Salvador MJ, Shotan A, Silversides CK, Skouby SO, Stein JI, Tornos P, Vejlstrup N,

Walker F, Warnes C. ESC Guidelines on the management of cardio-vascular diseases during pregnancy: the Task Force on the Management of Cardiovascular Diseases during Pregnancy of the European Society of Cardiology (ESC). Eur Heart J. 2011;32:3147–97.

Roos-Hesselink JW, Ruys TP, Stein JI, Thilen U, Webb GD, Niwa K, Kaemmerer H, Baumgartner H, Budts W, Maggioni AP, Tavazzi L, Taha N, Johnson MR, Hall R, Investigators R. Outcome of pregnancy in patients with structural or ischaemic heart disease: results of a registry of the European Society of Cardiology. Eur Heart J. 2013;34:657–65.

Sliwa K, Fett J, Elkayam U. Peripartum cardiomyopathy. Lancet. 2006a;368:687–93.

Sliwa K, Forster O, Libhaber E, Fett JD, Sundstrom JB, Hilfiker-Kleiner D, Ansari AA. Peripartum cardiomyopathy: inflammatory markers as predictors of outcome in 100 prospectively studied patients. Eur Heart J. 2006b;27:441–6.

Sliwa K, Blauwet L, Tibazarwa K, Libhaber E, Smedema JP, Becker A, McMurray J, Yamac H, Labidi S, Struhman I, Hilfiker-Kleiner D. Evaluation of bromocriptine in the treatment of acute severe peripartum cardiomyopathy: a proof-of-concept pilot study. Circulation. 2010a;121:1465–73.

Sliwa K, Hilfiker-Kleiner D, Petrie M, Mebazaa A, Pieske B, Buchmann E, Regitz-Zagrosek V, Schaufelberger M, Tavazzi B, van Veldhuisen DJ, Watkins H, Shah AJ, Seferovic PM, Elkayam U, Pankuweit S, Papp Z, Mouquet F, McMurray J. Current state of knowledge on aetiology, diagnosis, management, and therapy of peripartum cardiomyopathy: a position statement from the Heart Failure Association of the European Society of Cardiology Working Group on Peripartum Cardiomyopathy. Eur Heart J. 2010b;12:767–78.

Soma-Pillay P, MacDonald AP, Mathivha TM, Bakker JL, Mackintosh MO. Cardiac disease in pregnancy: a 4-year audit at Pretoria Academic Hospital. S Afr Med J. 2008;98:553–6.

Spirito P, Autore C. Management of hypertrophic cardiomyopathy. BMJ. 2006;332:1251–5.

Walenta K, Schwarz V, Schirmer S, Kindemann I, Friedrich E, Solomayer E, Sliwa K, Labidi S, Hilfiker-Kleiner D, Bohm M. Circulating microparticles as indicators of peripartum cardiomyopathy. Eur Heart J. 2012;33(12):1469–79.

Management of Coronary Artery Disease and Arrhythmias

Annemien E. van den Bosch, Titia P.E. Ruys, and Jolien W. Roos-Hesselink

Introduction

Although coronary artery disease is seldom encountered in women of childbearing age (16–45 years of age), the consequences of coronary disease are considerable, especially in pregnant women. Acute coronary syndrome (ACS) occurring in pregnancy can have devastating effects on mother and child. ACS in pregnancy has other causes than in the non-pregnant state. In the review of Roth and Elkayam only 40 % of the cases (41 of 103 patients) were caused by coronary artery stenosis (Roth and Elkayam 2008). Other causes were thrombus (in 8 % of cases), coronary artery dissection (27 %) and vascular spasm (2 %); normal coronary arteries were found in 13 % of the patients (Roth and Elkayam 2008). Pregnancy has shown to increase the risk of ACS three- to fourfold (James et al. 2006). Between 1991 and 2000 the overall incidence of pregnancy related ACS was reported to be 2.7 per 100,000 deliveries (Ladner et al. 2005). A decade later James et al. published on risk factors for ACS during pregnancy and reported an incidence of 6.2 per 100,000 deliveries

A.E. van den Bosch, MD, PhD • T.P.E. Ruys, MD
J.W. Roos-Hesselink, MD, PhD (✉)
Department of Cardiology, Thorax Center, Erasmus Medical Center, 's-Gravendijkwal 230, Rotterdam 3015 CE, The Netherlands
e-mail: j.roos@erasmusmc.nl

K. Sliwa, J. Anthony (eds.), *Cardiac Drugs in Pregnancy*, 53
Current Cardiovascular Therapy,
DOI 10.1007/978-1-4471-5472-3_4,
© Springer-Verlag London 2014

between 2000 and 2002 (James et al. 2006). The rising incidence can be explained in three ways: firstly improved diagnostic tests, especially troponin assessment, have resulted in more women with acute chest pain being diagnosed with ACS; secondly, an increase in known cardiovascular risk factors is seen in the pregnant population and finally, maternal age has increased in the Western World (Ventura et al. 2004). The most important risk factors for ACS during pregnancy are hypertension and maternal age (Cecchini et al. 2010). In addition to cardiovascular risk factors, a few obstetric risk factors for ACS during pregnancy have been discovered. The most important is multiparity; others include: a history of preeclampsia, post-partum haemorrhage, transfusions and post-partum infections (Ladner et al. 2005).

Adequate management of patients with coronary artery disease in pregnancy is of the utmost importance if survival rates are to improve.

A detailed knowledge of the normal physiological changes during pregnancy, labour and the postpartum period is essential for doctors looking after pregnant women with heart disease. The normal physiological changes of pregnancy alter the absorption, distribution and clearance of medications. There is a well-known increase in cardiac output and glomerular filtration rate during pregnancy, as well as a significantly increased volume of distribution for most drugs (Dawes and Chowienczyk 2001). The vast majority of oral medications also pass fairly freely through the placenta, thereby posing a potential risk to the developing fetus. Drugs used to treat coronary artery disease and arrhythmias fall into a few general categories including anticoagulants, cardiac glycosides, anti-anginals, angiotensin-converting enzyme inhibitors & angiotensin receptor-blockers. Some of these medications have more than one indication.

Preconception Counselling

Ideally all women of reproductive age with cardiac disease should undergo thorough evaluation before becoming pregnant. This evaluation should focus on identifying and quantifying the risk to the mother and her unborn child. During pre-pregnancy counselling life expectancy and ethical aspects of parenthood should also be discussed. Risk stratification is made to inform the patient of possible complications during pregnancy. Not only should the influence of pregnancy on the cardiac condition be considered, but the influence of the cardiac condition on the pregnancy outcome must also be discussed. These include the higher incidence of hypertension, preeclampsia, arrhythmias and thrombotic complications. Medication used for treatment during pregnancy is also of concern to the cardiologist, obstetrical care providers and patients. Many patients are under the mistaken belief that if they become pregnant they should stop their medications (Koren et al. 1998). Women and their care providers must weigh the risks and benefits of using each individual medication during pregnancy. In some instances, withholding the medication may be the best option, in others a 'safer' alternative medication(s) may be substituted, while in some cases continuation of the medication is advised, if necessary with dose adjustment. Preconception counselling for all women with coronary artery disease is therefore mandatory.

Medication for Coronary Artery Disease in Pregnancy

Beta-Blocking Agents

Beta-adrenergic receptor antagonists remain a cornerstone in the therapy of all stages of ischemic heart disease. Beta-blockade is standard therapy for effort angina, mixed effort and rest angina, and unstable angina. Beta blockers also decrease mortality in acute phase myocardial infarction and in the post infarct period. Today, a multitude of beta-blockers are available and can differ in their beta-1 and beta-2 receptor affinity, lipid solubility and intrinsic sympathomimetic activity. Beta-1 blockade reduces the oxygen demand of the heart by reducing the cardiac output by decreasing heart rate, while Beta-2 blockade causes constriction of airway smooth muscle and increases systemic vascular resistance (Magee 2001). Based on available human data, beta-blockers do not appear to be teratogenic. Beta-blockers cross the placenta and there has been some concern that they may cause neonatal bradycardia as well as transient hypoglycaemia and lower birth weight (Magee et al. 2001). In particular, Atenolol has been associated with intrauterine growth restriction (IUGR) (Butters et al. 1990). Reduced fetal growth is related to increased vascular resistance in the mother and fetus, and is a function of the length of drug exposure (von Dadelszen et al. 2000). The other beta-blockers are weakly associated with IUGR and have been used widely during pregnancy for various cardiac conditions.

Nitrate

In 1933 Sir Thomas Lewis held that the effect of amyl nitrite was probably due mainly to its powerful dilatation of the coronary vessels, rather than to its effect in lowering the blood pressure. As time went on, the important role of nitrate-induced venodilatation was recognized. This venous dilation causes a reduction in cardiac preload and (to a lesser degree) cardiac afterload. Nitroglycerin has been used for obstetrical reasons during pregnancy, such as preterm labour, with no adverse effects (Schleussner et al. 2003). Therefore, nitrates can safely be used during pregnancy, but hypotension may occur. The pre-eminent role for nitrates in pregnancy, however, is probably found in the pharmacologic management of congestive heart failure due to myocardial dysfunction (in conjunction with hydralazine), given the contraindication to the use of ACE inhibitors and ARBs prior to delivery. Nitroprusside is another nitrate option for acute afterload reduction (Shoemaker and Meyers 1984). This parenteral antihypertensive is very potent but poses the potential risk of cyanide accumulation and toxicity in the mother and the fetus following prolonged use.

Calcium Channel Blockers

Calcium channel blockers act chiefly by vasodilatation and reduction of the peripheral vascular resistance and against coronary spasm. They remain among the most commonly used agents in the treatment of hypertension and angina. Calcium channel blockers are a heterogeneous group of drugs that can chemically be classified into dihydropyridines and nondihydropyridines. Dihydropyridines, such as nifedipine and amlodipine, act predominately on the vasculature leading to smooth muscle relaxation and vasodilation. Nondihyropyridine calcium channel blockers (verapamil and diltiazem) act primarily on the heart and are often used to treat arrhythmias in pregnancy. Both classes of calcium channel blockers produce direct arterial vasodilation by inhibiting the influx of calcium through channels in smooth muscle. Nifedipine is used frequently to treat hypertension in pregnancy, as well as preterm labor. There have been no teratogenic risks associated with the use of nifedipine in pregnancy (Magee et al. 1996; Brown et al. 2002; Papatsonis et al. 2001). Amlodipine has been used less frequently during pregnancy, with very limited published data. A recent small case series was reassuring and there have been no animal studies showing that it is teratogenic or harmful to the fetus; however, amlodipine is not the first choice in the treatment of coronary artery disease, until there are more published human data available (Wagner et al. 1990; Briggs and Yaffe 2007).

Statins

Blood lipids are no longer a cardiologic curiosity; they form an essential step in the assessment of coronary artery disease for both primary and secondary prevention. Statins are the most commonly used drugs and shown to be very effective in reducing LDL cholesterol while increasing HDL cholesterol. They are competitive inhibitors of HMG CoA reductase, which is the rate-limiting step in cholesterol biosynthesis. Although statins have been identified as potential teratogens on the basis of theoretical considerations and small animal series, the available evidence is far from conclusive. Epidemiological data collected to date suggest that statins are not major teratogens (Kazmin et al. 2007). Based on the limited available human data regarding the use of statins, however, these agents are not recommended for use in pregnancy (Taguchi et al. 2008). In particularly high-risk women (i.e. recent MI or uncontrolled hyperlipidemia), the use of statins during pregnancy might be considered on an individual basis.

Acetylsalicylic Acid

Acetylsalicylic acid (ASA) is an antiplatelet agent, which irreversibly acetylates cyclooxygenase and activity is not restored until new platelets are formed. It has been shown that ASA (<100 mg/day) can be used safely during pregnancy (Czeizel and Rockenbauer 2000). A recent meta-analysis found no overall increase in the risk of congenital anomalies if aspirin was used in the first trimester, but there was a small increase in the risk of fetal gastroschisis (Kozer et al. 2002). Other studies showed no increase in the risk of maternal or fetal bleeding, nor placental abruption, with the use of low-dose ASA during pregnancy (Coomarasamy et al. 2003; Rotchell et al. 1998).

Thienopyridine

Ticlopidine and clopidogrel are thienopyridine derivates that irreversibly inhibit the binding of ADP to its receptor on the platelets, thereby preventing the transformation of the glycoprotein IIb/IIIa receptor into its active form. Thienopyridine derivates are used in patients with acute coronary syndromes and in patients with stents from percutaneous coronary interventions. There is very limited data on the use of these agents in pregnancy, but published cases are generally reassuring and the drugs do not appear to be teratogenic in animal studies (Briggs and Yaffe 2007; Al-Aqeedi and Al-Nabti 2008). The benefits of using thienopyridine derivates in a given high-risk pregnant woman (i.e., recent myocardial infarction with coronary stent) are likely to outweigh the potential fetal risks. Therefore, thienopyridine in pregnancy might be considered in high-risk cases.

Glycoprotein IIb/IIIa Receptor Antagonists

Glycoprotein IIb/IIIa inhibitors are frequently used during percutaneous coronary intervention (angioplasty with or without intracoronary stent placement). They work by preventing platelet aggregation and thrombus formation. There is very limited experience with the use of Glycoprotein IIb/IIIa receptor antagonists in pregnancy. Only a few case reports are documented in which patients received IIb/IIIa receptor antagonists after coronary stenting for an acute coronary syndrome during pregnancy. In these cases, no complications or adverse fetal outcomes were noted (Chow et al. 1998). These agents might be considered for use in pregnancy in high-risk clinical circumstances, but, in general, should be avoided, especially shortly before delivery.

The use of angiotensin-converting enzyme inhibitors & angiotensin receptor-blockers and antigoagulants in pregnancy will be discussed in another chapter of this book.

Table 1 gives an overview of the most common used medication for coronary heart disease and recommendations in pregnancy. In summary, low dose aspirin, beta blockade and nitrates can be continued during pregnancy. The safety of clopidogrel is unknown. In individual cases with recent (drug eluting) stent placement, continuation should be considered. ACE inhibitors and ARBs are advised to stopped in all patients or in the pre-conception clinic or immediately when pregnancy is diagnosed. Generally, statins should be stopped, however, in an individual patient with very high cholesterol, continuation may be considered.

TABLE I Drugs for coronary heart disease in pregnancy

Drugs	FDA	Listed complications	Transfer to breast milk
Atenolol	D	Intrauterine growth restriction and premature birth	Yes
Other beta-blockers	C	Low birth weight, hypoglycemia, and bradycardia in the fetus	Yes
Acetylsalicylic acid (ASA)	B	Low-dose aspirin is safe (large database)	Yes, but well-tolerated
Calcium channel antagonists	C	Diltiazem: an increase in major birth defects has been reported	Yes
Clopidogrel	C	The benefits of using clopidogrel in some high-risk pregnancies may outweigh the potential fetal risk	Unknown
Nitrates	B	Careful titration is advised to avoid maternal hypotension	Unknown
Statins	X	Animal studies demonstrated increased skeletal abnormalities, fetal and neonatal mortality.	Unknown

Percutaneous Intervention (PCI) or Coronary Artery Bypass Surgery

There is only limited information available on PCI during pregnancy. However, pregnancy is not a contraindication for PCI and since PCI is the primary treatment for non-pregnant STEMI (ST Elevation Myocardial Infarction) patients, more and more cases of stenting during pregnancy are published. With PCI as a treatment modality during pregnancy, mortality from ACS has dropped. In the first review of Roth and Elkayam in 1996 only 2 % had PCI, whereas in their second review 40 % had a PCI, all with bare metal stenting (Roth and Elkayam 1996, 2008). The preference for bare metal stenting is based on the requirement of dual anti-platelet treatment around the delivery and the lack of experience with this regime in pregnancy.

Since pregnant women are excluded from most clinical trials, no randomised controlled trials have been performed on thrombolytic therapy, PCI or CABG in the pregnancy. However, thrombotic therapy is considered to be relatively contraindicated in patient with ACS because of the risk of bleeding complications. In stroke, pulmonary embolism and mechanical heart valve thrombosis there is some clinical experience with several strategies such as tPA, urokinase and streptokinase. This medication does not cross the utero-placental barrier (Leonhardt et al. 2006). Maternal and fetal outcomes were favourable, but complications, such as maternal haemorrhage, fetal loss, abruptio placentae, preterm delivery and post partum haemorrhage have been reported in up to 10 % of cases with a maternal mortality rate of 1.2 % (Turrentine et al. 1995; Garvey et al. 1998).

Very limited data is available on coronary artery bypass grafting (CABG) during pregnancy and no conclusion concerning the safety of the mother and the unborn child can be made. In normal non-pregnant patients with ischemic heart disease CABG is used when multiple vessels or the left main coronary artery are involved (Nallamothu et al. 2005). In the case study of Roth and Elkayam ten patients were described who underwent CABG, of which seven were due to coronary artery dissection, in these cases one fetal death and one late maternal death were reported (Garvey et al. 1998; Roth and Elkayam 2008). If CABG is necessary for the management of the mother, it is advised to perform the CABG in the second trimester of pregnancy.

Delivery

Planning delivery should be the task of a multidisciplinary team consisting of at least an obstetrician, anaesthesiologist and cardiologist. The delivery should be postponed if possible for at least 2 or 3 weeks after ACS to allow adequate healing (Presbitero et al. 2009). The mode of delivery depends on the maternal hemodynamic situation and obstetric factors. Women with adequate cardiac output may tolerate induction of labour and vaginal delivery. Vaginal delivery can lead to fluctuations in blood pressure, especially if labour is pro-longed. Assisted vaginal delivery (by vacuum or forceps extraction) is recommended in high-risk women to avoid excessive maternal efforts and prolonged labour (Roth and Elkayam 2008). Adequate pain relief is very important, but epidural anaesthesia is contraindicated when the patient is on antithrombotic or anticoagulant treatment. As an alternative, narcotic analgesia can be used to reduce anxiety and pain. Vaginal delivery with a shortened second stage of labour and adequate pain relief can be safe and is preferred to caesarean section, especially as blood loss is lower. However, caesarean section is the preferred mode of delivery in patients with cardiac instability. During caesarean delivery, the blood pressure can be controlled, stress and pain relieved and a stable environment created. However, caesarean section has been associated with a higher risk of venous thrombo-embolism, infection and peripartum haemorrhage. In some cases general anaesthesia will be necessary with some risk of complications (Deneux-Tharaux et al. 2006). In addition, blood loss during caesarean section has been shown to be about twice as high as during vaginal delivery.

Breastfeeding

The effects of breast-feeding on maternal cardiovascular function are caused by circulating hormones. High levels of oxytocin circulate through the body. In the study of

Mezzacappa cardiac output during breastfeeding was found to be higher than in bottle-feeding mothers. They describe a decrease in heart rate and a slight increase in systolic blood pressure during the first minutes of breast-feeding (Mezzacappa et al. 2001). The fluctuations in blood pressure may be dangerous in severely symptomatic patients and bottle-feeding should be considered (Light et al. 2000).

Arrhythmias

Arrhythmias in pregnancy are common and may cause concern for the wellbeing of both the mother and child. The arrhythmias may be a recurrence of a previously diagnosed arrhythmia or the first presentation in a woman with known structural heart disease. In most cases, however, no previous history of heart disease is known, and the new occurrence of a cardiac problem can give rise to considerable anxiety. The majority of arrhythmias occurring during pregnancy are benign, and simply troublesome. Reassurance and advice about appropriate actions during symptomatic episodes are usually all that is required. In the remaining minority of cases, judicious use of antiarrhythmic drugs will lead to a safe and successful outcome for both mother and baby (Newstead-Angel and Gibson 2009). The major concern regarding the use of antiarrhythmic drugs is their potential adverse effects on the fetus. All antiarrhythmic drugs should be regarded as potentially toxic to the fetus.

Mechanism of Arrhythmia

The cardiovascular system undergoes significant changes in adaptation to pregnancy, including an increase in heart rate and cardiac output, reduced systemic resistance increased plasma catecholamine concentrations and adrenergic receptor sensitivity, atrial stretch and increased end-diastolic volumes due to intravascular volume expansion, as well as hormonal and emotional changes. A combination of these and the heightened visceral awareness experienced in pregnancy may lead a woman to seek advice on symptoms that are within the normal range and may otherwise have been ignored. Being pregnant is unlikely to generate a new arrhythmia, however, premature extra systolic beats are often seen during pregnancy.

Management of Specific Arrhythmias

Table 2 summaries the drug of choice for specific arrhythmias.

Supraventricular Tachycardia (SVT)

The drug of choice is partly dependent upon the SVT being treated. Atrioventricular nodal re-entry tachycardia (AVNRT) and atrioventricular re-entry tachycardia (AVRT) involving an accessory pathway can be terminated by vagal manoeuvres or if that fails, an intravenous bolus of adenosine can be administered until the desired response is achieved (Elkayam and Goodwin 1995). Intra-venous metoprolol is recommended if adenosine fails to terminate a tachycardia. Prophylactic antiarrhythmic medication should be used only if symptoms are intolerable or the arrhythmia causes haemodynamic instability. Digoxin or a selective beta-blocker (metoprolol) are the first-line drugs, followed by sotalol, or propafenone (Blomstrom-Lundqvist et al. 2003). AV nodal blocking agents should not be used in patients with manifest pre-excitation on resting ECG. Catheter ablation should be considered only in special cases if necessary during pregnancy.

Atrial Fibrillation and Flutter

Atrial fibrillation and flutter are uncommon in pregnancy and are most commonly associated with congenital or valvular

TABLE 2 Drugs for management of specific arrhythmias: to use or to avoid

Arrhythmia	Preferred medication	Avoid	Comments
Supraventricular tachycardia	Adenosine Metoprolol Digoxine Verapamil Sotalol Procainamide	Dispyramide Propafenone	β-blockade is often effective at suppressing ventricular ectopy and arrhythmias. Lidocaine followed by proacainamide is suggested for sustained ventricular arrhythmias. In refractory cases, amiodarone or placement of an ICD may be considered
Atrial fibrillation	Digoxin Metoprolol Verapamil Sotalol Fleicainide	Amiodarone	β-blockers, digoxin or verapamil may be used to slow the ventricular rate. Restoration of sinus rhythm is desirable (to avoid need for anticoagulation) and may be attempted with sotalol, procainamide, flecainide or electrical cardioversion.
Ventricular tachycardia	Metoprolol Procainamide Lidocaine	Amiodarone	β-blockade is often effective at suppressing ventricular ectopy and arrhythmias. Lidocaine followed by proacainamide is suggested for sustained ventricular arrhythmias.

heart disease as well as metabolic disturbances such as thyrotoxicosis or electrolyte imbalance. A rapid ventricular response to these arrhythmias can lead to serious haemodynamic consequences for both mother and fetus. Diagnosis and treatment of the underlying condition is therefore the first priority. Electrical cardioversion should be performed in the case of haemodynamic instability. In haemodynamically stable patients, pharmacological termination of the atrial or AF can be considered. Intravenous ibutilide or flecainide are usually effective, but experience during pregnancy is very limited (Kockova et al. 2007).

When rate control is recommended, the ventricular rate can be controlled with AV nodal blocking drugs including digoxin, beta-blockers and non-dihydropyridine calcium channel antagonist (verapamil, diltiazem) (Fuster et al. 2006). Prophylactic antiarrhythmic drugs (sotalol, flecainide or propafenone) may be considered in the cases of severe symptoms despite rate-controlling drugs. Flecainide and propafenone should be combined with AV nodal blocking agents. Mexiletine and amiodarone are contra-indicated in pregnancy with the exception of an acute setting or as last resort (European Society of Gynecology et al. 2011).

The recommendation in respect of anticoagulation in atrial fibrillation and flutter will be discussed in another chapter.

Ventricular Tachycardia (VT)

Life-threatening ventricular arrhythmias are uncommon during pregnancy. Rapid VT causes hypotension, reduced myocardial coronary perfusion and subendocardial ischaemia, an unstable situation that may degenerate into ventricular fibrillation. In healthy patients, idiopathic right ventricular tachycardia (VT) originating from the right ventricular outflow tract is the most frequent type in pregnancy and should be treated using either verapamil or beta-blocking agents. The drugs should be used as prophylaxis only if the VT is associated with severe symptoms or haemodynamic compromise (Nakagawa et al. 2004).

Ventricular tachycardia in the presence of structural heart disease is associated with a significant risk of sudden death and requires emergency treatment. For acute treatment of VT with haemodynamic instability, immediate cardioversion, which seems safe in all phases of pregnancy, is recommended. Prophylactic therapy with a cardioselective beta-blocker, such as metoprolol, may be effective (European Society of Gynecology et al. 2011). Sotalol or Class Ic antiarrhythmic drugs may be considered in the absence of structural heart disease.

Antiarrhythmic Drugs in Pregnancy

The decision to treat a woman depends upon the type of arrhythmia, frequency, duration and tolerability of the arrhythmia. It is a balance between the benefit of arrhythmia reduction or termination and the maternal and fetal side effects of any drug treatment. The greatest risk to the fetus is during organogenesis and this is complete by the end of the first trimester. The smallest recommended dose should be used initially and be accompanied by regular monitoring of the maternal and fetal condition. An overview of medications used in the treatment of arrhythmia, including their pharmacokinetics, mechanism of action, indications, safety and effectiveness in pregnancy is set out in Table 3.

Beta-Blockers

Metoprolol is a common choice for treating tachyarrhythmias and available pregnancy data are reassuring. Propranolol also has good safety data regarding its use in pregnancy, but is a non-selective beta-blocking agent and offers no clear advantage over metoprolol for most cardiac indications.

TABLE 3 Drugs for arrhythmias in pregnancy

Drugs	FDA	Listed complications	Transfer to breast milk
Adenosine	C	Pregnant women may respond to lower doses due to a reduction in adenosine deaminase	No
Atropine	C	Insufficient data	Yes, small amount
Amiodarone (Class III)	D	If prolonged use; fetal hypo- and hyperthyroidism, goitre, IUGR, prematurity	Yes, avoid during breast feeding
Beta-blockers	C	IUGR, bradycardia, apnoea, hypoglycaemia, hyperbilirubinaemia	Yes
Digoxin	C	Miscarriage and fetal death in toxicity	Yes, small amount
Calcium channel antagonists	C	Skeletal abnormalities, IUGR, fetal death Verapamil: rapid injection may cause maternal ↓ BP and fetal distress.	Unknown
Disopyramide (Class IA)	C	Premature uterine contractions	Yes
Flecainide (Class IC)	C	Insufficient data but no reported significant complications. Concerns over its pro-arrhythmic potential in fetus have limited its use in past	Yes
Lidocaine (Class IB)	C	Fetal distress may occur in fetal toxicity	Yes
Quinidine (Class IA)	C	Rarely, mild uterine contractions, premature labour, neonatal thrombocytopenia, fetal VIIIn damage	Yes

TABLE 3 (continued)

Drugs	FDA	Listed complications	Transfer to breast milk
Procainamide (Class IA)	C	Chronic use may be associated with lupus-like syndrome, gastrointestinal disturbance, hypotension, agranulocytosis	Yes
Propafenone (Class IC)	C	Insufficient data	Unknown
Mexiletine (Class IB)	C	Fetal bradycardia	Yes
Sotalol (Class III)	B	Transient fetal bradycardia an hypoglycemia	Yes

BP blood pressure, *IUGR* intrauterine growth restriction, *SVT* supraventricular tachyarrhythmia

Calcium Channel Blockers

The nondihydropyridine calcium channel blockers (verapamil and diltiazem) slow conduction through the AV node and increase the refractory period of nodal tissue. Verapamil and diltiazem are similar in their electrophysiological properties and are used to treat arrhythmias in pregnancy. There is very limited published data regarding their safety and effectiveness. Verapamil in pregnancy has more published experience and does not appear to pose a significant teratogenic risk (Magee et al. 1996).

Sotalol

Sotalol is a class III anti-arrhythmic and combines beta-blockade with potassium channel blockade, causing prolongation of the refractory period of atrial, AV nodal, bypass tract and ventricular tissue. It is known that sotalol crosses the placenta. Limited published data do not show a teratogenic risk. As with other beta-blockers, some data have shown a risk of reduced placental weight and/or IUGR (O'Hare et al. 1980; Wagner et al. 1990). As Sotalol can also prolong the QT interval of the mother, posing a risk of proarrhythmia (mainly torsades de pointes), this medication should be restricted to use in cases where there is clearly a need for an antiarrhythmic agent (i.e., significant ventricular arrhythmias or recurrent atrial fibrillation) and where the maternal benefits are likely to outweigh these risks.

Amiodarone

Amiodarone is a unique "wide-spectrum" antiarrhythmic agent, chiefly class III, but also with powerful class I activity and ancillary class II an IV activity. It is a very potent antiarrhythmic drug in the general cardiac population, but its use in pregnancy is problematic. Amiodarone is associated with an increased risk of prematurity, fetal bradycardia and fetal/neonatal hypothyroidism (given its high iodine content). There have been congenital abnormalities reported in neonates exposed in the first trimester (Joglar and Page 1999; James 2001). It also poses a small risk of maternal proarrhythmia due to prolonged QT syndrome. Amiodarone is, therefore, only recommended for use in pregnancy in the setting of life-threatening conditions where other agents have failed.

Procainamide

Procainamide is a class Ia antiarrhythmic drug. It prolongs the action potential and the effective refractory period. It may be effective for both atrial and ventricular arrhythmias. Procainamide is often well tolerated and useful in the management of maternal and fetal arrhythmias. It may be administered orally, or intravenously in the management of an acute arrhythmia (James 2001; Joglar and Page 1999). Long-term use of procainamide can result in a lupus-like syndrome but it is well-tolerated for short-term use with a favourable adverse effect profile. Dose adjustments may be needed over the course of pregnancy.

Adenosine

Adenosine is very effective in the treatment of acute supraventricular tachycardia as it causes a transient conduction block in the atrioventricular node. It has been used safely and effectively in the acute treatment of supraventricular tachyarrhythmias during pregnancy with no significant adverse effects on the fetus (Kanai et al. 1996; Elkayam and Goodwin 1995). Minor maternal adverse effects include transient bradycardia and dyspnoea. It can also induce bronchospasm and is, therefore, not recommended in patients with asthma.

Digoxin

Digoxin has a long and safe history for use during pregnancy. Its main actions are through vagal-mediated slowing and blockade of atrioventricular conduction, as well as a mild prokinetic effect on the heart. Digoxin freely crosses the placenta and has been used for the treatment of fetal arrhythmias. The main issue with the use of digoxin in pregnancy is its effectiveness. The digoxin levels may decrease by 50 % during pregnancy due to increased renal clearance and an increase in dose is often required. In addition, levels must be monitored and dose adjustments made, particularly in patients with renal insufficiency. Digoxin will continue to have a role in the treatment of maternal and fetal arrhythmias as well as an adjunctive role in heart failure in pregnancy.

Table 2 gives an overview of the most commonly used medication for coronary heart disease and recommendations for use during pregnancy.

DC Cardioversion

DC cardioversion is safe in all stages of pregnancy; because the amount of current reaching the fetus is small. There is a small risk of inducing a fetal arrhythmia. The fetus needs to be carefully monitored during the cardioversion procedure.

Implantable Cardioverter-Defibrillators

The presence of an implantable cardioverter-defibrillators (ICD) is not itself a contraindication to future pregnancy and women with ICDs have had successful pregnancies with good fetal outcomes. Treatment with an ICD should also be considered during pregnancy to protect the mother's life in those at high risk of sudden cardiac death (European Society of Gynecology et al. 2011). One study reported a series of 44 pregnant women with an ICD implant in situ and found no increase in either device or treatment complications during pregnancy, nor any increase in the number of shocks the women received compared to preconception (Natale et al. 1997). In addition to standard ICD management, after each therapy, fetal monitoring is advised.

Conclusion

Pregnancy may unmask latent cardiac disease or may lead to a new onset of maternal cardiovascular disease or arrhythmias. Morbidity and mortality due to coronary artery disease in pregnancy appears to have increased during the last 30 years. Women with known ischemic heart disease or a history of arrhythmias with or without underlying heart disease need careful preconception counselling, as well as multidisciplinary management during pregnancy. Medication for coronary artery disease or arrhythmias in pregnancy is of concern to both care providers and patients. The ever-expanding pool of cardiac medication and devices needs careful monitoring during pregnancy and regular updating. Caution is required in respect of utility and risks when interventions are used during pregnancy.

US FDA Risk Classification in Pregnancy

The US Department of Health and Human Service have published this classification. (Source: *Drug information for the*

Heath Care Professional; USDPI Vol 1, Micromedex 23rd edn. 01.01.2003). The classification consists of category A (safest) to X (known danger – do not use). The following categories are used for drugs during pregnancy and breastfeeding.

Category A: controlled studies show no risk

Controlled studies in women fail to demonstrate a risk to the fetus in the first trimester, there is no evidence of a risk in later trimester and, therefore, the possibility of fetal harm appears remote

Category B: no evidence of risk in humans

Either animal reproduction studies have not demonstrated a fetal risk but there are no controlled studies in pregnant women, or animal reproduction studies have shown an adverse effect (other than a decrease in fertility) that was not confirmed in controlled studies in women in the first trimester (and there is no evidence of a risk in later trimester)

Category C: risk cannot be ruled out

Either studies in animals have revealed adverse effects on the fetus (teratogenic) or appropriate animal data are not available. Drugs should be given only if the potential benefit justifies the potential risk to the fetus

Category D: positive evidence of risk

There is positive evidence of human fetal risk, but the benefits from use in pregnant women may be acceptable despite the risk (e.g., if the drug is needed in a life-threatening situation or for a serious disease for which safer drugs cannot be used or are ineffective). There will be an appropriate statement in the 'warnings' section of the labeling

Category X: contraindicated in pregnancy

Studies in animals or human beings have demonstrated fetal abnormalities or there is evidence of fetal risk based on human experience, or both, and the risk of the use of the drug in pregnant women clearly outweighs any possible benefit. The drug is contraindicated in women who are or may be pregnant

References

Al-Aqeedi RF, Al-Nabti AD. Drug-eluting stent implantation for acute myocardial infarction during pregnancy with use of glycoprotein IIb/IIIa inhibitor, aspirin and clopidogrel. J Invasive Cardiol. 2008;20:E146–9.

Blomstrom-Lundqvist C, Scheinman MM, Aliot EM, Alpert JS, Calkins H, Camm AJ, Campbell WB, Haines DE, Kuck KH, Lerman BB, Miller DD, Shaeffer CW, Stevenson WG, Tomaselli GF, Antman EM, Smith Jr SC, Alpert JS, Faxon DP, Fuster V, Gibbons RJ, Gregoratos G, Hiratzka LF, Hunt SA, Jacobs AK, Russell Jr RO, Priori SG, Blanc JJ, Budaj A, Burgos EF, Cowie M, Deckers JW, Garcia MA, Klein WW, Lekakis J, Lindahl B, Mazzotta G, Morais JC, Oto A, Smiseth O, Trappe HJ, European Society of Cardiology Committee, N.-H. R. S. ACC/AHA/ESC guidelines for the management of patients with supraventricular arrhythmias – executive summary. A report of the American college of cardiology/American heart association task force on practice guidelines and the European society of cardiology committee for practice guidelines (writing committee to develop guidelines for the management of patients with supraventricular arrhythmias) developed in collaboration with NASPE-Heart Rhythm Society. J Am Coll Cardiol. 2003;42:1493–531.

Briggs G, Yaffe F. Drugs in pregnancy and lactation: a reference guide to fetal and neonatal risk. 8th ed. Philadelphia: Lippincott, Williams and Wilkins; 2007.

Brown CS, Ling FW, Wan JY, Pilla AA. Efficacy of static magnetic field therapy in chronic pelvic pain: a double-blind pilot study. Am J Obstet Gynecol. 2002;187:1581–7.

Butters L, Kennedy S, Rubin PC. Atenolol in essential hypertension during pregnancy. BMJ. 1990;301:587–9.

Cecchini M, Sassi F, Lauer JA, Lee YY, Guajardo-Barron V, Chisholm D. Tackling of unhealthy diets, physical inactivity, and obesity: health effects and cost-effectiveness. Lancet. 2010;376:1775–84.

Chow T, Galvin J, McGovern B. Antiarrhythmic drug therapy in pregnancy and lactation. Am J Cardiol. 1998;82:58I–62I.

Coomarasamy A, Honest H, Papaioannou S, Gee H, Khan KS. Aspirin for prevention of preeclampsia in women with historical risk factors: a systematic review. Obstet Gynecol. 2003;101:1319–32.

Czeizel AE, Rockenbauer M. A population-based case-control teratologic study of oral oxytetracycline treatment during pregnancy. Eur J Obstet Gynecol Reprod Biol. 2000;88:27–33.

Dawes M, Chowienczyk PJ. Drugs in pregnancy. Pharmacokinetics in pregnancy. Best Pract Res Clin Obstet Gynaecol. 2001;15:819–26.

Deneux-Tharaux C, Carmona E, Bouvier-Colle MH, Breart G. Postpartum maternal mortality and cesarean delivery. Obstet Gynecol. 2006;108:541–8.

Elkayam U, Goodwin TM. Adenosine therapy for supraventricular tachycardia during pregnancy. Am J Cardiol. 1995;75:521–3.

European Society of Gynecology, Association for European Paediatric Cardiology, German Society for Gender Medicine, Regitz-Zagrosek V, Blomstrom Lundqvist C, Borghi C, Cifkova R, Ferreira R, Foidart JM, Gibbs JS, Gohlke-Baerwolf C, Gorenek B, Iung B, Kirby M, Maas, AH, Morais J, Nihoyannopoulos P, Pieper PG, Presbitero P, Roos-Hesselink JW, Schaufelberger M, Seeland U, Torracca L, ESC Committee for Practice Guidelines. ESC guidelines on the management of cardiovascular diseases during pregnancy: the Task Force on the Management of Cardiovascular Diseases during Pregnancy of the European Society of Cardiology (ESC). Eur Heart J. 2011;32:3147–97.

Fuster V, Ryden LE, Cannom DS, Crijns HJ, Curtis AB, Ellenbogen KA, Halperin JL, Le Heuzey JY, Kay GN, Lowe JE, Olsson SB, Prystowsky EN, Tamargo JL, Wann S, Smith Jr SC, Jacobs AK, Adams CD, Anderson JL, Antman EM, Hunt SA, Nishimura R, Ornato JP, Page RL, Riegel B, Priori SG, Blanc JJ, Budaj A, Camm AJ, Dean V, Deckers JW, Despres C, Dickstein K, Lekakis J, McGregor K, Metra M, Morais J, Osterspey A, Zamorano JL. ACC/AHA/ESC 2006 guidelines for the management of patients with atrial fibrillation – executive summary: a report of the American College of Cardiology/American Heart Association Task Force on Practice Guidelines and the European Society of Cardiology Committee for Practice Guidelines (Writing Committee to Revise the 2001 Guidelines for the Management of Patients With Atrial Fibrillation). J Am Coll Cardiol. 2006;48:854–906.

Garvey P, Elovitz M, Landsberger EJ. Aortic dissection and myocardial infarction in a pregnant patient with Turner syndrome. Obstet Gynecol. 1998;91:864.

James PR. Drugs in pregnancy. Cardiovascular disease. Best Pract Res Clin Obstet Gynaecol. 2001;15:903–11.

James AH, Jamison MG, Biswas MS, Brancazio LR, Swamy GK, Myers ER. Acute myocardial infarction in pregnancy: a United States population-based study. Circulation. 2006;113:1564–71.

Joglar JA, Page RL. Treatment of cardiac arrhythmias during pregnancy: safety considerations. Drug Saf. 1999;20:85–94.

Kanai M, Shimizu M, Shiozawa T, Ashida T, Sawaki S, Sasaki Y, Fujii S. Use of intravenous adenosine triphosphate (ATP) to terminate supraventricular tachycardia in a pregnant woman with Wolff-Parkinson-White syndrome. J Obstet Gynaecol Res. 1996;22:95–9.

Kazmin A, Garcia-Bournissen F, Koren G. Risks of statin use during pregnancy: a systematic review. J Obstet Gynaecol Can. 2007;29: 906–8.

Kockova R, Kocka V, Kiernan T, Fahy GJ. Ibutilide-induced cardioversion of atrial fibrillation during pregnancy. J Cardiovasc Electrophysiol. 2007;18:545–7.

Koren G, Pastuszak A, Ito S. Drugs in pregnancy. N Engl J Med. 1998;338:1128–37.

Kozer E, Nikfar S, Costei A, Boskovic R, Nulman I, Koren G. Aspirin consumption during the first trimester of pregnancy and congenital anomalies: a meta-analysis. Am J Obstet Gynecol. 2002;187:1623–30.

Ladner HE, Danielsen B, Gilbert WM. Acute myocardial infarction in pregnancy and the puerperium: a population-based study. Obstet Gynecol. 2005;105:480–4.

Leonhardt G, Gaul C, Nietsch HH, Buerke M, Schleussner E. Thrombolytic therapy in pregnancy. J Thromb Thrombolysis. 2006;21: 271–6.

Light KC, Smith TE, Johns JM, Brownley KA, Hofheimer JA, Amico JA. Oxytocin responsivity in mothers of infants: a preliminary study of relationships with blood pressure during laboratory stress and normal ambulatory activity. Health Psychol. 2000;19:560–7.

Magee LA. Drugs in pregnancy. Antihypertensives. Best Pract Res Clin Obstet Gynaecol. 2001;15:827–45.

Magee LA, Schick B, Donnenfeld AE, Sage SR, Conover B, Cook L, McElhatton PR, Schmidt MA, Koren G. The safety of calcium channel blockers in human pregnancy: a prospective, multicenter cohort study. Am J Obstet Gynecol. 1996;174:823–8.

Magee LA, Bull SB, Koren G, Logan A. The generalizability of trial data; a comparison of beta-blocker trial participants with a prospective cohort of women taking beta-blockers in pregnancy. Eur J Obstet Gynecol Reprod Biol. 2001;94:205–10.

Mezzacappa ES, Kelsey RM, Myers MM, Katkin ES. Breast-feeding and maternal cardiovascular function. Psychophysiology. 2001;38:988–97.

Nakagawa M, Katou S, Ichinose M, Nobe S, Yonemochi H, Miyakawa I, Saikawa T. Characteristics of new-onset ventricular arrhythmias in pregnancy. J Electrocardiol. 2004;37:47–53.

Nallamothu BK, Saint M, Saint S, Mukherjee D. Clinical problem-solving. Double jeopardy. N Engl J Med. 2005;353:75–80.

Natale A, Davidson T, Geiger MJ, Newby K. Implantable cardioverter-defibrillators and pregnancy: a safe combination? Circulation. 1997; 96:2808–12.

Newstead-Angel J, Gibson PS. Cardiac drug use in pregnancy: safety, effectiveness and obstetric implications. Expert Rev Cardiovasc Ther. 2009;7:1569–80.

O'Hare MF, Murnaghan GA, Russell CJ, Leahey WJ, Varma MP, McDevitt DG. Sotalol as a hypotensive agent in pregnancy. Br J Obstet Gynaecol. 1980;87:814–20.

Papatsonis DN, Lok CA, Bos JM, Geijn HP, Dekker GA. Calcium channel blockers in the management of preterm labor and hypertension in pregnancy. Eur J Obstet Gynecol Reprod Biol. 2001;97: 122–40.

Presbitero PBG, Groot C, Roos-Hesselink J. Pregnancy and heart disease. In: ESC textbook of cardiovascular medicine. Oxford: Oxford University Press; 2009.

Rotchell YE, Cruickshank JK, Gay MP, Griffiths J, Stewart A, Farrell B, Ayers S, Hennis A, Grant A, Duley L, Collins R. Barbados Low Dose Aspirin Study in Pregnancy (BLASP): a randomised trial for the prevention of pre-eclampsia and its complications. Br J Obstet Gynaecol. 1998;105:286–92.

Roth A, Elkayam U. Acute myocardial infarction associated with pregnancy. Ann Intern Med. 1996;125:751–62.

Roth A, Elkayam U. Acute myocardial infarction associated with pregnancy. J Am Coll Cardiol. 2008;52:171–80.

Schleussner E, Moller A, Gross W, Kahler C, Moller U, Richter S, Seewald HJ. Maternal and fetal side effects of tocolysis using transdermal nitroglycerin or intravenous fenoterol combined with magnesium sulfate. Eur J Obstet Gynecol Reprod Biol. 2003;106:14–9.

Shoemaker CT, Meyers M. Sodium nitroprusside for control of severe hypertensive disease of pregnancy: a case report and discussion of potential toxicity. Am J Obstet Gynecol. 1984;149:171–3.

Taguchi N, Rubin ET, Hosokawa A, Choi J, Ying AY, Moretti ME, Koren G, Ito S. Prenatal exposure to HMG-CoA reductase inhibitors: effects on fetal and neonatal outcomes. Reprod Toxicol. 2008;26: 175–7.

Turrentine MA, Braems G, Ramirez MM. Use of thrombolytics for the treatment of thromboembolic disease during pregnancy. Obstet Gynecol Surv. 1995;50:534–41.

Ventura SJ, Abma JC, Mosher WD, Henshaw S. Estimated pregnancy rates for the United States, 1990–2000: an update. Natl Vital Stat Rep. 2004;52:1–9.

von Dadelszen P, Ornstein MP, Bull SB, Logan AG, Koren G, Magee LA. Fall in mean arterial pressure and fetal growth restriction in pregnancy hypertension: a meta-analysis. Lancet. 2000;355:87–92.

Wagner X, Jouglard J, Moulin M, Miller AM, Petitjean J, Pisapia A. Coadministration of flecainide acetate and sotalol during pregnancy: lack of teratogenic effects, passage across the placenta, and excretion in human breast milk. Am Heart J. 1990;119:700–2.

Anticoagulation in Pregnancy

Vera Regitz-Zagrosek, Christa Gohlke-Baerwolf, Bernard Iung, and Petronella G. Pieper

Abbreviations

EF   Ejection fraction
INR   International normalized ratio
LMWH   Low molecular weight heparin
UFH   Unfractioned heparin

─────────

V. Regitz-Zagrosek, MD (✉)
Charité, University Medicine Berlin, Institute of Gender in
Medicine (GiM), Charité Campus Mitte, Hessische Str. 3-4,
Berlin 10115, Germany

University Medicine Berlin, Center for Cardiovascular
Research (CCR), Berlin, Germany
e-mail: vera.regitz-zagrosek@charite.de; http://gender.charite.de

C. Gohlke-Baerwolf, MD
Department of Cardiology, Heart Center Bad Krozingen,
Bad Krozingen, Germany

B. Iung, MD
Cardiology Department, AP-HP, Bichat Hospital, Paris, France

University Paris Diderot, Sorbonne Paris Cité, Paris, France

P.G. Pieper, MD
Department of Cardiology, University Medical Center Groningen,
University of Groningen, Groningen, The Netherlands

K. Sliwa, J. Anthony (eds.), *Cardiac Drugs in Pregnancy*,   79
Current Cardiovascular Therapy,
DOI 10.1007/978-1-4471-5472-3_5,
© Springer-Verlag London 2014

Introduction

In pregnant women, anticoagulation is needed for women with mechanical valves, for women who are at increased risk of venous thrombembolism, those who have cardiomyopathies and severely impaired ejection fraction (EF), for high-risk patients with atrial fibrillation, those who have acute coronary syndromes and for some patients with congenital heart disease. The most frequently used drugs are Vitamin K antagonists, heparins, clopidogrel, and acetyl salicylic acid. They differ in the level of protection and risk they bear for the mother and her fetus and their precise use varies according to the specific indication. Both the indications and drugs have been discussed in the guidelines of the European Society of Cardiology on the management of cardiovascular diseases in pregnancy and were recently reviewed in European Heart Journal ((Regitz-Zagrosek et al. 2011) and Current Problems in Cardiology). The present chapter is based on these publications.

The Drugs

The most frequently used anticoagulants in pregnancy are heparins, vitamin K antagonists and acetylsalicylic acid used as an anti-aggregant drug. With few exceptions, they have rarely been studied in prospective trials (McLintock et al. 2009; Barbour et al. 2004; Schaefer et al. 2006). Knowledge is mainly based on observational studies and retrospective analysis of registries (Sillesen et al. 2011). Experiences with unplanned and planned exposure to drugs in pregnancy are collected in two large databases: www.embryotox.de and www.safefetus.com. Accordingly drugs have been classified by FDA into categories A-X in relation to pregnancy (Table 1). The European Society of Cardiology guidelines on Management of cardiovascular diseases in Pregnancy list drugs with their FDA classification, their reported adverse effects for mother, fetus and the newborn. They also specify each drug's placenta permeability and transfer into breast milk.

TABLE 1 FDA categories for classification of drugs in pregnancy

Pregnancy Category A	Adequate and well-controlled human studies have failed to demonstrate a risk to the fetus in the first trimester of pregnancy (and there is no evidence of risk in later trimesters).
Pregnancy Category B	Animal reproduction studies have failed to demonstrate a risk to the fetus and there are no adequate and well-controlled studies in pregnant women OR Animal studies have shown an adverse effect, but adequate and well-controlled studies in pregnant women have failed to demonstrate a risk to the fetus in any trimester.
Pregnancy Category C	Animal reproduction studies have shown an adverse effect on the fetus and there are no adequate and well-controlled studies in humans, but potential benefits may warrant use of the drug in pregnant women despite potential risks.
Pregnancy Category D	There is positive evidence of human fetal risk based on adverse reaction data from investigational or marketing experience or studies in humans, but potential benefits may warrant use of the drug in pregnant women despite potential risks.
Pregnancy Category X	Studies in animals or humans have demonstrated fetal abnormalities and/or there is positive evidence of human fetal risk based on adverse reaction data from investigational or marketing experience, and the risks involved in use of the drug in pregnant women clearly outweigh potential benefits.
Pregnancy Category N	FDA has not classified this drug.

Heparin is a well-studied drug in pregnancy. The most common adverse effects observed include osteoporosis and thrombocytopenia in the mother, if the drug is used for longer periods (Regitz-Zagrosek et al. 2011). These adverse effects are significantly less frequent if low molecular weight heparin (LMWH) is used. Heparins do not cross the placenta and are not transferred to breast milk. They are classified by FDA as B.

Warfarin, acenocoumarol and phenprocoumon are known to induce coumarin-embryopathies, probably in a dose dependent manner. They will cross the placenta and are transferred to breast milk in low amounts (10 %, well tolerated as inactive metabolites). Warfarin and acenocoumarol are classified by FDA into category D.

The newer anticoagulant Danaparoid (with a heparin like action) is classified category B by FDA. No teratogenic effects were found in animal studies or in approximately 80 reported human cases (www.embryotox.de). It may be used as an alternative to heparins if these are contraindicated – for example in Heparin induced thrombocytopenia.

The newer anticoagulant drugs have not been evaluated in pregnancy and are therefore not recommended in pregnant patients. This applies to Dabigatran, a direct thrombin inhibitor, and the Factor Xa-inhibitors Rivaroxaban, Apixaban and Fondaparinux.

All these new drugs cross the placental barrier in varying degrees and are also therefore not recommended.

For acetyl salicylic acid large datasets are available that do not describe any teratogenic effects. It crosses the placenta and is transferred to the breast milk, but appears to be well tolerated. It is classified category B by FDA. For the platelet inhibitor Clopidogrel, no teratogenity was found in rat and mouse studies and in more than 30 documented human cases (www.embrytox.de). Transfer to breast milk is unknown. Clopidogrel has recently been upgraded from category C to B by the FDA classification. The use of more recent antiplatelet drugs (prasugrel, ticagrelor), bivalirudin and glycoprotein IIb/IIIa inhibitors is not recommended during pregnancy because of insufficient safety data (Regitz-Zagrosek et al. 2011).

Mechanical Valves

Pregnancy in patients with mechanical valves is associated with an increased risk of valve thrombosis, of haemorrhagic complications, and adverse perinatal outcome. The character and magnitude of the maternal and associated fetal risk depends largely on the anticoagulation regimen used during pregnancy and the quality of anticoagulation control.

The procoagulant mechanisms associated with pregnancy contribute to the markedly increased risk of valve thrombosis in pregnant women. In a large review this risk was 3.9 % with oral anticoagulants throughout pregnancy, 9.2 % when unfractionated heparin (UFH) was used in the first trimester and oral anticoagulants in the second and third trimester, and 33 % with UFH throughout pregnancy (Chan et al. 2000). Maternal death occurred in these groups in 2, 4, and 15 %, respectively, and was usually related to valve thrombosis (Chan et al. 2000). A review of recent literature confirmed the low risk of valve thrombosis with oral anticoagulants throughout pregnancy (2.4 %, 7/287 pregnancies) compared to UFH in the first trimester (10.3 %, 16/156 pregnancies) (Abildgaard et al. 2009). The risk is probably lower with adequate dosing and is also dependant on type and position of the mechanical valve as well as on additional patient-related risk factors.

UFH throughout pregnancy is additionally associated with thrombocytopenia and osteoporosis. LMWHs are also associated with the risk of valve thrombosis (Oran et al. 2004; Elkayam et al. 2004). The risk is lower, but still present, with dose adjusting according to anti-Xa levels (Oran et al. 2004; McLintock et al. 2009; Quinn et al. 2009; Yinon et al. 2009; Abildgaard et al. 2009). In 111 pregnancies in which LMWH with dose adjustment according to anti-Xa levels were used throughout pregnancy, valve thrombosis occurred in 9 % (Oran et al. 2004). Too lower target anti-Xa levels or poor compliance probably contributed to valve thrombosis in all but one pregnancy. A review reported lower frequency of valve thrombosis with LMWH in the first trimester only, but in a small patient group (3.6 %, 2/56 pregnancies) (Abildgaard et al. 2009).

The use of LMWH during pregnancy in women with mechanical prostheses is still controversial because evidence is scarce. Unresolved questions concern optimal anti-Xa levels, the importance of peak versus pre-dose levels and the best time intervals for anti-Xa monitoring. Studies are urgently needed.

There is a marked increase in dose requirement during pregnancy to keep the anti- Xa levels in the therapeutic range, (Barbour et al. 2004; Quinn et al. 2009) because of increased volume of distribution and increased renal clearance. Therefore regular monitoring of anti-Xa levels is necessary. It has been demonstrated that pre-dose anti-Xa levels are often subtherapeutic when peak levels are between 0.8 and 1.2 U/ml (Barbour et al. 2004; Friedrich and Hameed 2010). Even when predose anti-Xa level monitoring and more frequent dosing lead to higher pre-dose levels combined with lower peak levels, there are no data available to show that this approach achieves a stable, consistent therapeutic intensity of anticoagulation and will prevent valve thrombosis and bleeding (Yinon et al. 2009; Barbour et al. 2004; Friedrich and Hameed 2010).

Current evidence indicates that oral anticoagulants throughout pregnancy, under strict international normalized ratio control, are the safest regimen for the mother (Chan et al. 2000; Abildgaard et al. 2009; Sillesen et al. 2011). However adequate randomized studies that compare different regimens are not available. The superiority of either UFH or LMWH in the first trimester is unproven though a recent review suggests higher efficacy of LMWH (Abildgaard et al. 2009). However the only randomized study comparing weight adjusted doses of LMWH (enoxaparin) with warfarin and initial UFH in pregnant women was prematurely terminated after the occurrence of valve thrombosis in two of seven women on LMWH (HIP-CAT study) (Oran et al. 2004; Elkayam et al. 2004) No LMWH is officially approved (labelled) for pregnant women with mechanical valves in any country.

All anticoagulation regimens carry an increased risk of miscarriage and of haemorrhagic complications, including retroplacental bleeding leading to premature birth and fetal death (Elkayam and Bitar 2005; Chan et al. 2000; McLintock et al. 2009; Oran et al. 2004; Quinn et al. 2009; Yinon et al. 2009). Comparison between studies is however impaired by reporting differences. Oral anticoagulants cross the placenta and their use in the first trimester can result in embryopathy in 0.0–10 % of cases (Schaefer et al. 2006; Vitale et al. 1999; Chan et al. 2000). UFH and LMWH do not cross the placenta and embryopathy does not occur. Substitution of oral anticoagulants with UFH in weeks 6–12 nearly eliminates the risk of embryopathy. The incidence of embryopathy was low (2.6 %) in a small series when warfarin dose was <5 mg and 8 % when warfarin dose was >5 mg daily (Cotrufo et al. 2002; Vitale et al. 1999; Sillesen et al. 2011). The dose-dependency was confirmed in several recent studies (Cotrufo et al. 2002; Vitale et al. 1999; Sillesen et al. 2011) however not in all (McLintock 2013). Major central nervous system abnormalities occur in 1 % of children when oral anticoagulants are used in the first trimester (van Driel et al. 2002). A low risk of minor central nervous system abnormalities and intracranial bleeding exists with oral anticoagulants outside the first trimester only (van Driel et al. 2002) whereby the intensity of anticoagulation and its control plays a significant role. Vaginal delivery while the mother is on oral anticoagulants is contraindicated because of the risk of fetal intracranial bleeding.

Individualized Management

Pre-pregnancy evaluation should include assessment of symptoms and echocardiographic evaluation of ventricular function, as well as prosthetic and native valve function. Type and position of the prosthetic valve(s) as well as history of valve thrombosis should be taken into account. The advantages and disadvantages of different anticoagulation regimens should be discussed extensively. The mother and her partner must understand that according to current evidence oral anticoagulants are the most effective regimen to prevent valve thrombosis, and therefore the safest regimen for her; those risks that put the mothers life in jeopardy will also jeopardize the survival of the baby. On the other hand the risk of embryopathy and fetal hemorrhage also needs discussion.

Compliance with prior anticoagulant therapy should be considered and the management of the regimen that is chosen should be planned in detail. The effectiveness of the anticoagulation regimen should be monitored weekly and clinical follow-up including echocardiography should be performed monthly.

Individual Drug Therapy

The main goal of anticoagulation therapy in pregnant women with mechanical valves is to prevent the occurrence of valve thrombosis and its lethal consequences for both mother and fetus. The following recommendations should be seen in this perspective. The class of recommendations based on the wording used is explained in Table 2.

Oral anticoagulants should be continued until pregnancy is achieved.

UFH or LMWH throughout pregnancy is not recommended because of the high risk of valve thrombosis with these regimens in combination with low fetal risk with oral anticoagulants in the second and third trimester-. Continuation of oral anticoagulants throughout pregnancy should be considered when warfarin dose is <5 mg daily (or phenprocoumon <3 mg or acenocoumarol <2 mg daily) because the risk of embryopathy is low, while oral anticoagulants are in large series the most effective regimen to prevent valve thrombosis (Chan et al. 2000; Sillesen et al. 2011). After full disclosure to the pregnant woman that oral anticoagulants throughout pregnancy are the safest regimen for her and that low dose coumarin therapy carries an embryopathy risk of less than 3 %, discontinuation of oral anticoagulants and a switch to UFH or LMWH between pregnancy weeks 6 and 12 (under strict dose control and supervision) may be considered. When a higher-dose oral anticoagulants are required, discontinuation of oral anticoagulants between weeks 6 and 12 and replacement by adjusted-dose UFH (activated partial thromboplastin time ≥2 times the control, in high risk patients applied as intravenous infusion) or LMWH (twice daily with dose adjustment according to weight and according to anti-Xa

TABLE 2 Classes of recommendation

Classes of recommendations	Definition	Suggested wording to use
Class I	Evidence and/or general agreement that a given treatment or procedure is beneficial, useful, effective.	Is recommended/is indicated
Class II	Conflicting evidence and/or a divergence of opinion about the usefulness/efficacy of the given treatment or procedure.	
Class IIa	Weight of evidence/opinion is in favour of usefulness/efficacy.	Should be considered
Class IIb	Usefulness/efficacy is less well established by evidence/opinion.	May be considered
Class III	Evidence or general agreement that the given treatment or procedure is not useful/effective, and in some cases may be harmful.	Is not recommended

levels) should be considered. The anti-Xa level should be maintained between 0.8 and 1.2 U/ml, determined 4–6 h after dosing (Butchart et al. 2005; Regitz-Zagrosek et al. 2011). The European Society of Cardiology task force (Regitz-Zagrosek et al. 2011) advises weekly control of peak anti-Xa levels because of the need for increasing dosages of LMWH during pregnancy (Vahanian et al. 2012; Barbour et al. 2004; Bonow et al. 2006; Abildgaard et al. 2009; Quinn et al. 2009).

The importance of also monitoring the pre-dose level of anti-Xa, and the necessity to maintain this level above 0.6 IU/ml, has been insufficiently studied, particularly in relation to thrombo-embolic events and bleeding and no firm recommendations can be made. The starting dose for LMWH is 1 mg/kg bodyweight if enoxaparin is chosen and 100 IU/kg for dalteparin, given twice daily subcutaneously. The dose should be adjusted according to increasing weight during pregnancy (Lebaudy et al. 2008) and anti-Xa levels. The European Society of Cardiology task force does not recommend the addition of acetylsalicylic acid to this regimen because there are no data to prove its efficacy and safety in pregnant women. The use of LMWH in the first trimester is limited by several factors including the scarcity of data about its efficacy (Abildgaard et al. 2009) and safety, uncertainties concerning the optimal dosing to prevent both valve thrombosis and bleeding, and the variable availability of anti-Xa level testing.

Irrespective of the regimen used, the effect of the anticoagulants should be monitored very carefully, and in the case of oral anticoagulants the international normalized ratio (INR) should be determined at weekly intervals. The intensity of the INR should be chosen according to the type and location of the prosthetic valve, according to present guidelines (Vahanian et al. 2012). Intense education about anticoagulation and self-monitoring of anticoagulation in suitable patients is recommended. In cases where UFH is used, once a stable activated partial thromboplastin time has been achieved, the aPTT should be monitored weekly by 4–6 h after starting the first dose, aiming for prolongation of the aPTT by ≥ 2 times the control.

Diagnosis and Management of Valve Thrombosis

When a woman with a mechanical valve presents with dyspnoea and/or an embolic event, immediate transthoracic echocardiography is indicated to search for valve thrombosis, usually followed by transoesophageal echocardiography. Fluoroscopy can be performed with limited fetal risk. The management of valve thrombosis is similar to the management in non-pregnant patients. This includes optimizing anticoagulation using intravenous heparin and resumption of oral anticoagulation in non-critically ill patients with recent sub-therapeutic anticoagulation. Surgery is indicated when anticoagulation fails and for critically ill patients with obstructive thrombosis (Vahanian et al. 2012). Most fibrinolytic agents do not cross the placenta, but the risk of embolization (10 %) and of retroplacental bleeding leading to obstetric haemorrhage is a concern and experience in pregnancy is limited. Fibrinolysis should be applied in critically ill patients when surgery is not immediately available. Because fetal loss is high with surgery, fibrinolysis may be considered instead of surgery in non-critically ill patients when anticoagulation fails. Fibrinolysis is the therapy of choice in right-sided prosthetic valve thrombosis (Vahanian et al. 2012). The mother should be informed about the risks (see Table 2).

Venous Thromboembolism

Pregnancy and the puerperium are associated with a five times higher risk of venous thromboembolism than in the general female population of childbearing age. Venous thromboembolism complicates about 0.05–0.20 % of all pregnancies (Liu et al. 2009; Heit et al. 2005; O'Connor et al. 2010; Rutherford and Phelan 1991; Sullivan et al. 2004). Venous thromboembolism encompasses pulmonary embolism and deep vein thrombosis. Pulmonary embolism is the third most common cause of direct maternal death in the UK occurring in 0.70/100,000 maternities (Wilkinson and Trustees and Medical Advisers 2011). The case fatality rate is 3.5 % (Knight 2008).

The presence of risk factors contributes to an increased risk of venous thromboembolism during pregnancy and the puerperium. Seventy nine percent of women dying from an antenatal pulmonary embolism in the UK had identifiable risk factors (CEMACH 2008; Knight 2008). The most significant risk factors for venous thromboembolism in pregnancy are a prior history of unprovoked deep vein thrombosis or pulmonary embolism (Marik and Plante 2008) and thrombophilias.

In the recent CMACE- study (Wilkinson and Trustees and Medical Advisers 2011) 88 % of women dying of pulmonary embolism had risk factors, but being overweight or obese were the most important risk factors. The identification of risk factors influences the choice of preventive strategies. All women should undergo a documented assessment of risk factors for venous thromboembolism before pregnancy or in early pregnancy. Based on type and number of risk factors present in the individual patient three risk groups can be identified (high, intermediate and low-risk groups) and preventive measures applied accordingly.

Patients at high risk are those with previous recurrent venous thromboembolism and previous unprovoked or oestrogen related venous thromboembolism or a single previous venous thromboembolism associated with a thrombophilic condition or a family history of thromboembolic disease.

Patients with intermediate risk are those with three or more risk factors other than those listed as high-risk factors. These include: pregnancy with medical co-morbidities, maternal age >35 years, obesity (body mass index >30 kg/m$^{2)}$, hyperemesis and dehydration, smoking, gross varicose veins, and obstetric factors like pre-eclampsia, ovarian hyperstimulation syndrome, multiple pregnancy, caesarean section, prolonged labour (> 24 h) and peripartum hemorrhage (>1 l or transfusion). Transient risk factors are current systemic infection, immobility, any surgical procedure in pregnancy or <6 weeks post-partum.

Patients at low risk are those with less than three risk factors, except for overweight and obesity, which was shown to be an important risk factor of its own. However the influence of single risk factors other than those included in the high risk group is not known.

LMWH has become the drug of choice for the prevention of venous thromboembolism in pregnant women. It causes less bone loss than UFH and the osteoporotic fracture rate is lower (0.04 % of pregnant women treated with LMWH) (Greer and Nelson-Piercy 2005; Bates et al. 2008; Royal College of Obstetricians and Gynecologists 2009).

The dose of LMWH for thromboprophylaxis is based on bodyweight. However, previous recommended doses are mostly based on studies in non-pregnant patients, and there are no studies available on the optimal doses in women who are obese or puerperal (Bates et al. 2008). Although the incidence of venous thromboembolism decreased recently, particularly in obese patients a significant residual risk of venous thromboembolism remains (Wilkinson and Trustees and Medical Advisers 2011). It is therefore suggested, that women of high risk should receive a prophylactic dose of LMWH that is half of the therapeutic dose, weight adjusted, applied twice daily (e.g. Enoxaparin of 0.5 mg/kg body weight twice daily or Dalteparin 50 units/kg 12 hourly) (Regitz-Zagrosek et al. 2011) and studies should be conducted in these patients.

Acute Deep Vein Thrombosis

Deep vein thrombosis (DVT) is characterized by leg swelling, which is a frequent finding in pregnancy. Since deep vein thrombosis is left sided in over 85 % of cases, due to compression of the left iliac vein by the right iliac artery and the gravid uterus, swelling of the left leg is specifically suspicious. A clinical decision rule has been suggested based upon three variables: if the suspected DVT does not affect the left leg presentation, if the calf circumference difference is <2 cm and if the presentation was later than the first trimester combined with negative ultrasound examination of the legs, the negative predictive value is 100 % (95 % CI 95.8–100 %) (Chan et al. 2009). This clinical decision-rule needs validation in prospective studies.

D-Dimer levels increase physiologically with each trimester. In one study the mean preconception D-dimer concentration was 0.43 (SD 0.49) mg/L, and rose in the first, second, and third trimester to 0.58 mg/L (SD 0.36), 0.83 (SD 0.46) mg/L, and 1.16 (SD 0.57) mg/L, respectively, indicating a 39 % relative increase in D-dimer concentration for each trimester compared with the previous one (Kline et al. 2005).

Thus a positive D-dimer test based on the conventional cut-off level is not necessarily indicative of DVT and new cut-off levels are needed. However, the degree of the pregnancy related increase in D-dimer levels rarely reaches levels which usually are associated with DVT. Therefore the ESC guidelines recommend that the diagnosis is made by determination of D-Dimer levels, respecting the physiologically increased levels and compression ultrasound leg vein imaging. Compression ultrasound leg vein imaging has a high sensitivity and specificity for proximal deep vein thrombosis. Serial compression ultrasonography with Doppler imaging of the iliac vein performed over a 7-day period excludes deep-vein thrombosis in symptomatic pregnant women (Chan et al. 2013).

Treatment in acute deep vein thrombosis is based on the use of therapeutic doses of LMWH. LMWH should be administered in a weight adjusted, twice daily regimen (see treatment of pulmonary embolism).

Pulmonary Embolism

Symptoms and signs of pulmonary embolism during pregnancy are the same as in the non-pregnant state (new onset dyspnoea, chest pain, tachycardia, haemoptysis and collapse). Clinical assessment of pulmonary embolism is however more difficult, because dyspnoea and tachycardia are not uncommon in normal pregnancy. A high index of suspicion is important for the timely diagnosis of venous thromboembolism. All pregnant women with signs and symptoms suggestive of venous thromboembolism, particularly dyspnoea of acute onset or worsening dyspnoea should have objective testing performed as expeditiously as it is the case in non-pregnant patients. According to the consensus of the European Society of Cardiology task force (Regitz-Zagrosek et al. 2011) D-dimer concentration should be measured in patients with suspected pulmonary embolism, followed by bilateral compression ultrasonography. If this is normal in the presence of negative

D-dimer levels then pulmonary embolism is unlikely and anti-coagulation with LMWH is not warranted.

In patients with suspected pulmonary embolism, positive D-dimer levels and positive compression ultrasonography, anticoagulation treatment is indicated. If D-dimer levels are elevated and compression ultrasonography is negative in patients with suspected pulmonary embolism, further testing is required. Computed tomography pulmonary angiography should be performed, when the diagnosis cannot be confirmed or excluded with the above discussed tools. In these patients it is preferred over ventilation–perfusion lung scanning for the diagnosis of pulmonary embolism (Torbicki et al. 2008). Both techniques are associated with fetal radiation exposure, with ventilation–perfusion lung scanning delivering a higher fetal dose of radiation than computed tomography pulmonary angiography. However, radiation doses are below the limit that is regarded as dangerous for the fetus (Torbicki et al. 2008; Winer-Muram et al. 2002).

LMWH has also become the drug of choice for the treatment of venous thromboembolism in pregnancy and puerperium. The efficacy and safety of several LMWH preparations was shown in a review of 2,777 pregnant women, treated for deep vein thrombosis or pulmonary embolism. The risk of recurrent venous thromboembolism with treatment doses of LMWH was 1.15 %. The observed rate of major bleeding was 1.98 %. Heparin – induced thrombocytopenia is markedly lower with LMWH than with UFH and so is heparin – induced osteoporosis (0.04 %) (Greer and Nelson-Piercy 2005). In clinically suspected deep vein thrombosis or pulmonary embolism treatment with LMWH should be given until the diagnosis is excluded by objective testing. The recommended therapeutic dose is calculated on bodyweight (e.g. Enoxaparin 1 mg/kg bodyweight twice daily, Dalteparin 100 IU/kg bodyweight twice daily) aiming for peak anti-Xa values (4–6 h post-dose) of 0.6–1.2 IU/ml (Bates et al. 2008). The necessity to monitor anti-Xa values regularly in patients with venous thromboembolism is still controversial. Whereas it is considered necessary in patients with mechanical valves in whom LMWH is used this is not so clear in patients with venous thromboembolism. Given the need for dose-increase as pregnancy progresses to maintain a certain therapeutic anti-Xa –level (Barbour et al. 2004; Friedrich and Hameed 2010) it seems reasonable to also determine anti-Xa levels during pregnancy in patients with venous thromboembolism. This appears particularly justified in view of the fact, that pulmonary embolism occurred in women receiving preventive doses of LMWH (Knight 2008). This topic also requires further studies. A simple guide is to adjust the dose according to increasing weight during pregnancy.

UFH also does not cross the placenta, but is associated with more thrombocytopenia, osteoporosis and more frequent dosing when given subcutaneously compared to LMWH. It is favoured in patients with renal failure and when urgent reversal of anticoagulation by protamine may be needed as well as in the acute treatment of massive pulmonary emboli. In patients with acute pulmonary embolism with haemodynamic compromise intravenous administration of UFH is recommended (loading dose of 80 units/kg, followed by a continuous intravenous infusion of 18 units/kg/h).

The activated partial thromboplastin time has to be determined 4–6 h after the loading dose, 6 h after any dose change and then at least daily when in the therapeutic range. The therapeutic target activated partial thromboplastin time ratio is usually 1.5–2.5 times the average laboratory control value. The dose is then titrated to achieve a therapeutic activated partial thromboplastin time, defined as the activated partial thromboplastin time that corresponds to an anti-Xa level of 0.3–0.7 IU/mL. After improvement in haemodynamics and stabilisation of the patient UFH can be switched to LMWH in therapeutic doses and maintained during pregnancy. LMWH should be switched to intravenous UFH at least 36 h before the induction of labour or caesarean delivery. UFH should be discontinued 4–6 h before anticipated delivery, and restarted 6 h after delivery if there are no bleeding complications. Neither UFH nor LWMH are found in breast milk in any significant amount and they do not represent a contraindication to breastfeeding.

Thrombolysis

Thrombolytics are considered to be relatively contraindicated during pregnancy and peripartum and should only be used in high risk patients with severe hypotension or shock (Torbicki et al. 2008). The risk of haemorrhage, mostly from the genital tract, is about 8 % (Turrentine et al. 1995). In about 200 reported patients, mostly streptokinase was used and more recently recombinant tissue plasminogen activator. Both thrombolytics do not cross the placenta in significant amounts. Fetal loss of 6 and 6 % preterm delivery were reported (Ahearn et al. 2002). Urokinase does cross the placenta and is therefore not primarily advised. There are very few studies on fondaparinux in pregnancy, one has shown minor transplacental passage of fondaparinux (Dempfle 2004). Because of the scarce data it should not be used in pregnancy.

In patients with recent pulmonary embolism, heparin treatment should be restarted 6 h after a vaginal birth and 12 h after a caesarean delivery, if no significant bleeding has occurred. Dose adjustments may be necessary because of decreases in blood volume and renal clearance. Vitamin K antagonists may be started on the second day after delivery and continued for at least 3–6 months (6 months if pulmonary embolism occurred late in pregnancy). The INR should be between 2 and 3 and needs regular monitoring, ideally once every 1–2 weeks. Vitamin K antagonists do not enter the breast milk in active forms and are safe for nursing mothers.

Cardiomyopathies and Heart Failure

The aetiology of cardiomyopathies occurring in association with pregnancy is diverse with acquired (peripartum cardiomyopathy, toxic cardiomyopathy) and inherited (hypertrophy cardiomyopathy, dilated cardiomyopathy, storage disease, etc.) forms of cardiomyopathy. Their incidence differs according to regions and the precise incidence in Europe is not known. However, mothers with cardiomyopathies have a high mortality during and after pregnancy (Sliwa et al. 2010). A thrombus in the left ventricle and associated embolic events are rare but dangerous complications of heart failure due to cardiomyopathies. The European Society of Cardiology guidelines on treatment of chronic heart failure recommend anticaoagulation with vitamin K antagonists for patients with very low ejection fraction; ventricular thrombi or atrial fibrillation (McMurray et al. 2012). Accordingly, pregnant women who have a dilated or peripartum cardiomyopathy together with atrial arrhythmias or ventricular thrombi should be anticoagulated using LMWH or Vitamin K antagonists according to stage of pregnancy, as discussed above. The newer anticoagulant agents (dabigatran, apixaban, fondaparinux) are not recommended because of lack of experience.

Care should be taken with anti-coagulation therapy in the immediate phase after delivery, but once the risk of obstetric haemorrhage has passed, it should be considered in patients with very low EF. Peripheral embolism including cerebral embolism and ventricular thrombi are especially frequent in peripartum cardiomyopathy patients (Sliwa et al. 2010). This is in part due to increased procoagulant activity in the peripartum phase (Brenner 2004).

In hypertrophic cardiomyopathy therapeutic anticoagulation with LMWH or Vitamin K antagonists is recommended for those with paroxysmal or persistent atrial fibrillation.

Atrial Fibrillation

Patients with valvular atrial fibrillation with either native or prosthetic valves require anticoagulation during pregnancy. For management of patients with prosthetic valves see above chapter on mechanical valves. Also in patients with native valves atrial fibrillation is associated with a high thromboembolic risk, particularly in patients with severe mitral stenosis. The occurrence of atrial fibrillation requires immediate anticoagulation with intravenous UFH, followed by LMWH in the first and last trimester and oral anticoagulants or LMWH for the second trimester. LMWH should be given in weight- adjusted therapeutic doses (twice daily) until 36 h prior to delivery. If oral anticoagulants are used, the INR can be kept between 2.0 and 2.5, thus minimizing the risk for the fetus.

The thromboembolic risk in non-valvular atrial fibrillation depends upon the presence of risk factors. Patients without structural heart disease or risk factors ("lone atrial fibrillation") have the lowest risk of thromboembolic events and do not require anticoagulation or antiplatelet therapy outside or during pregnancy; however, studies during pregnancy are not available. An increase in thromboembolic risk in non-valvular atrial fibrillation is assessed with the $CHADS_2$ criteria (Fuster et al. 2006) and the CHA_2DS_2VASC score (Camm et al. 2010) in non-pregnant patients. In these, oral anticoagulation is only beneficial when the thromboembolic risk is ≥ 4.0 events per 100 patient years (correlates to ≥ 2 risk points with the $CHADS_2$ score or 2 risk points with the CHA_2DS_2VASC score). The same considerations therefore apply to pregnant patients; thromboprophylaxis is recommended in patients with increased CHA_2DS_2VASC scores. The choice of the anticoagulant is made according to the stage of pregnancy. Vitamin K antagonists are recommended in most cases from the second trimester until 1 month before expected delivery (Camm et al. 2010). Subcutaneous administration of weight adjusted therapeutic doses of LMWH is recommended during the first trimester and during the last month of pregnancy. Not enough safety data are available for the newer anticoagulant agents in pregnancy (Dabigatran, Apixaban, Fondaparinux or Rivaroxaban). Either single or dual antiplatelet therapy (clopidogrel and acetylsalicylic acid) were not as effective as warfarin in high risk patients with atrial fibrillation (Healey et al. 2008; Camm et al. 2010).

Studies in non-pregnant older patients show that LMWH is effective and can be used if appropriate monitoring is available. Subcutaneous administration of weight adjusted therapeutic doses is recommended during the first trimester and during the last month of pregnancy.

For patients with atrial fibrillation duration <48 h and no thromboembolic risk factors, intravenous heparin or weight adjusted therapeutic dose LMWH may be considered pericardioversion, without the need for post-cardioversion oral anticoagulation. The indications for prophylactic antiarrhythmic drugs and anticoagulation relates to the presence of symptoms and the presence of risk factors for thromboembolism, respectively (Camm et al. 2012). In patients with risk factors for stroke or atrial fibrillation recurrence, antithrombotic treatment should be continued following cardioversion (Camm et al. 2012).

Acute Coronary Syndromes

Acute coronary syndromes in pregnancy may be an indication for use of antithrombotic agents in the context of percutaneous coronary intervention and stent implantation. Primary percutaneous coronary intervention is the preferred modality of reperfusion during pregnancy since it avoids potential hazards of thrombolysis and it is the only means to diagnose and treat spontaneous coronary dissection. Spontaneous coronary artery dissections are more prevalent among pregnant than non-pregnant women, occurring mainly around delivery or in the early postpartum period (Roth and Elkayam 2008). Stenting should favor the use of bare-metal stents with 3–4 weeks of dual antiplatelet therapy (Regitz-Zagrosek et al. 2011). UFH or LMWH is used during percutaneous coronary intervention and stopped after 24–48 h. Because of the relatively higher frequency of spontaneous coronary dissection in pregnancy, intravenous thrombolysis should be used only in women with ST-segment elevation ACS who cannot be treated with primary percutaneous coronary intervention. Recombinant tissue plasminogen activator does not cross the placenta but carries a bleeding risk, in particular retroplacental bleeding.

The use of antiplatelet agents is rarely indicated in pregnancy. It should be limited to the shortest duration possible, for example after stent implantation. In this case, Clopidogrel and aspirin should be used. The use of more recent antiplatelet drugs (prasugrel, ticagrelor), bivalirudin and glycoprotein IIb/IIIa inhibitors is not recommended during pregnancy (Regitz-Zagrosek et al. 2011).

Congenital Heart Disease

Anticoagulation therapy is an issue in pregnant women with congenital heart disease when they have mechanical valves, (paroxysmal) atrial fibrillation or flutter, or severely reduced ejection fraction. Women with pulmonary hypertension who have an indication for anticoagulation outside pregnancy should continue anticoagulation therapy during pregnancy (Regitz-Zagrosek et al. 2011). In women with pulmonary hypertension associated with intracardiac shunts, both the risk of thromboembolism and of bleeding are elevated. These women are prone to haemoptysis and thrombocytopenia. Therefore, the indication for anticoagulation should be carefully considered on an individual basis.

In women with the Fontan circulation, the risk of thromboembolism is considered high, especially in patients with an atriopulmonary connection. Therefore therapeutic anticoagulation should be considered.

In patients with congenital heart disease anticoagulation therapy is chosen dependant on the stage of pregnancy, with LMWH in the first trimester and the last month of pregnancy, while vitamin K antagonists can be used in the second and third trimester.

References

Abildgaard U, Sandset PM, Hammerstrom J, Gjestvang FT, Tveit A. Management of pregnant women with mechanical heart valve prosthesis: thromboprophylaxis with low molecular weight heparin. Thromb Res. 2009;124:262–7.

Ahearn GS, Hadjiliadis D, Govert JA, Tapson VF. Massive pulmonary embolism during pregnancy successfully treated with recombinant tissue plasminogen activator: a case report and review of treatment options. Arch Intern Med. 2002;162:1221–7.

Barbour LA, Oja JL, Schultz LK. A prospective trial that demonstrates that dalteparin requirements increase in pregnancy to maintain therapeutic levels of anticoagulation. Am J Obstet Gynecol. 2004;191: 1024–9.

Bates SM, Greer IA, Pabinger I, Sofaer S, Hirsh J. Venous thromboembolism, thrombophilia, antithrombotic therapy, and pregnancy: American College of Chest Physicians Evidence-Vased Clinical Practice Guidelines (8th edition). Chest. 2008;133:844S–86.

Bonow RO, Carabello BA, Chatterjee K, de Leon Jr AC, Faxon DP, Freed MD, Gaasch WH, Lytle BW, Nishimura RA, O'Gara PT, O'Rourke RA, Otto CM, Shah PM, Shanewise JS, Smith Jr SC, Jacobs AK, Adams CD, Anderson JL, Antman EM, Fuster V, Halperin JL, Hiratzka LF, Hunt SA, Lytle BW, Nishimura R, Page RL, Riegel B. ACC/AHA 2006 guidelines for the management of patients with valvular heart disease: a report of the American College of Cardiology/ American Heart Association Task Force on Practice Guidelines (writing Committee to Revise the 1998 guidelines for the management of patients with valvular heart disease) developed in collaboration with the Society of Cardiovascular Anesthesiologists endorsed by the Society for Cardiovascular Angiography and Interventions and the Society of Thoracic Surgeons. J Am Coll Cardiol. 2006;48:e1–148.

Brenner B. Haemostatic changes in pregnancy. Thromb Res. 2004; 114:409–14.

Butchart EG, Gohlke-Barwolf C, Antunes MJ, Tornos P, De Caterina R, Cormier B, Prendergast B, Iung B, Bjornstad H, Leport C, Hall RJ, Vahanian A. Recommendations for the management of patients after heart valve surgery. Eur Heart J. 2005;26:2463–71.

Camm AJ, Kirchhof P, Lip GY, Schotten U, Savelieva I, Ernst S, Van Gelder IC, Al-Attar N, Hindricks G, Prendergast B, Heidbuchel H, Alfieri O, Angelini A, Atar D, Colonna P, De Caterina R, De Sutter J, Goette A, Gorenek B, Heldal M, Hohloser SH, Kolh P, Le Heuzey JY, Ponikowski P, Rutten FH. Guidelines for the management of atrial fibrillation: the Task Force for the Management of Atrial Fibrillation of the European Society of Cardiology (ESC). Eur Heart J. 2010;31: 2369–429.

Camm AJ, Lip GY, De Caterina R, Savelieva I, Atar D, Hohnloser SH, Hindricks G, Kirchhof P, Guidelines, E. S. C. C. f. P., Bax JJ, Baumgartner H, Ceconi C, Dean V, Deaton C, Fagard R, Funck-Brentano C, Hasdai D, Hoes A, Kirchhof P, Knuuti J, Kolh P, McDonagh T, Moulin C, Popescu BA, Reiner Z, Sechtem U, Sirnes PA, Tendera M, Torbicki A, Vahanian A, Windecker S, Document R, Vardas P, Al-Attar N, Alfieri O, Angelini A, Blomstrom-Lundqvist C,

Colonna P, De Sutter J, Ernst S, Goette A, Gorenek B, Hatala R, Heidbuchel H, Heldal M, Kristensen SD, Kolh P, Le Heuzey JY, Mavrakis H, Mont L, Filardi PP, Ponikowski P, Prendergast B, Rutten FH, Schotten U, Van Gelder IC, Verheugt FW. 2012 focused update of the ESC Guidelines for the management of atrial fibrillation: an update of the 2010 ESC Guidelines for the management of atrial fibrillation. Developed with the special contribution of the European Heart Rhythm Association. Eur Heart J. 2012;33:2719–47.

CEMACH. CEMACH saving mothers' lives: reviewing maternal deaths to make motherhood safer — 2003–2005: the seventh report on confidential enquiries into maternal deaths in the United Kingdom. In: HEALTH, C. C. E. I. M. A. C., editor. London: Centre for Maternal and Child Enquiries; 2008.

Chan WS, Anand S, Ginsberg JS. Anticoagulation of pregnant women with mechanical heart valves: a systematic review of the literature. Arch Intern Med. 2000;160:191–6.

Chan WS, Lee A, Spencer FA, Crowther M, Rodger M, Ramsay T, Ginsberg JS. Predicting deep venous thrombosis in pregnancy: out in "LEFt" field? Ann Intern Med. 2009;151:85–92.

Chan WS, Spencer FA, Lee AY, Chunilal S, Douketis JD, Rodger M, Ginsberg JS. Safety of withholding anticoagulation in pregnant women with suspected deep vein thrombosis following negative serial compression ultrasound and iliac vein imaging. Can Med Assoc J. 2013;185:E194–200.

Cotrufo M, De Feo M, De Santo LS, Romano G, Della Corte A, Renzulli A, Gallo C. Risk of warfarin during pregnancy with mechanical valve prostheses. Obstet Gynecol. 2002;99:35–40.

Dempfle CE. Minor transplacental passage of fondaparinux in vivo. N Engl J Med. 2004;350:1914–5.

Elkayam U, Bitar F. Valvular heart disease and pregnancy: part II: prosthetic valves. J Am Coll Cardiol. 2005;46:403–10.

Elkayam U, Singh H, Irani A, Akhter MW. Anticoagulation in pregnant women with prosthetic heart valves. J Cardiovasc Pharmacol Ther. 2004;9:107–15.

Friedrich E, Hameed AB. Fluctuations in anti-factor Xa levels with therapeutic enoxaparin anticoagulation in pregnancy. J Perinatol. 2010;30: 253–7.

Fuster V, Ryden LE, Cannom DS, Crijns HJ, Curtis AB, Ellenbogen KA, Halperin JL, Le Heuzey JY, Kay GN, Lowe JE, Olsson SB, Prystowsky EN, Tamargo JL, Wann S. ACC/AHA/ESC 2006 guidelines for the management of patients with atrial fibrillation-executive summary: a report of the American College of Cardiology/American Heart Association Task Force on Practice Guidelines and the European Society of Cardiology Committee for Practice Guidelines (Writing Committee to Revise the 2001 Guidelines for the Management of Patients with Atrial Fibrillation). Eur Heart J. 2006;27:1979–2030.

Greer IA, Nelson-Piercy C. Low-molecular-weight heparins for throm-boprophylaxis and treatment of venous thromboembolism in preg-nancy: a systematic review of safety and efficacy. Blood. 2005;106: 401–7.

Healey JS, Hart RG, Pogue J, Pfeffer MA, Hohnloser SH, De Caterina R, Flaker G, Yusuf S, Connolly SJ. Risks and benefits of oral anticoagu-lation compared with clopidogrel plus aspirin in patients with atrial fibrillation according to stroke risk: the atrial fibrillation clopidogrel trial with irbesartan for prevention of vascular events (ACTIVE-W). Stroke. 2008;39:1482–6.

Heit JA, Kobbervig CE, James AH, Petterson TM, Bailey KR, Melton 3rd LJ. Trends in the incidence of venous thromboembolism during pregnancy or postpartum: a 30-year population-based study. Ann Intern Med. 2005;143:697–706.

Kline JA, Williams GW, Hernandez-Nino J. D-dimer concentrations in normal pregnancy: new diagnostic thresholds are needed. Clin Chem. 2005;51:825–9.

Knight M. Antenatal pulmonary embolism: risk factors, management and outcomes. BJOG. 2008;115:453–61.

Lebaudy C, Hulot JS, Amoura Z, Costedoat-Chalumeau N, Serreau R, Ankri A, Conard J, Cornet A, Dommergues M, Piette JC, Lechat P. Changes in enoxaparin pharmacokinetics during pregnancy and implications for antithrombotic therapeutic strategy. Clin Pharmacol Ther. 2008;84:370–7.

Liu S, Rouleau J, Joseph KS, Sauve R, Liston RM, Young D, Kramer MS. Epidemiology of pregnancy-associated venous thromboembolism: a population-based study in Canada. J Obstet Gynaecol Can. 2009;31:611–20.

Marik PE, Plante LA. Venous thromboembolic disease and pregnancy. N Engl J Med. 2008;359:2025–33.

McLintock C. Anticoagulant choices in pregnant women with mechani-cal heart valves: balancing maternal and fetal risks–the difference the dose makes. Thromb Res. 2013;131 Suppl 1:S8–10.

McLintock C, McCowan LM, North RA. Maternal complications and pregnancy outcome in women with mechanical prosthetic heart valves treated with enoxaparin. BJOG. 2009;116:1585–92.

McMurray JJ, Adamopoulos S, Anker SD, Auricchio A, Bohm M, Dickstein K, Falk V, Filippatos G, Fonseca C, Gomez-Sanchez MA, Jaarsma T, KoberL, Lip GY, Maggioni AP, Parkhomenko A, Pieske BM, Popescu BA, Ronnevik PK, Rutten FH, Schwitter J, Seferovic P, Stepinska J, Trindade PT, Voors AA, Zannad F, Zeiher A, Task Force for the D, Treatment of A, Chronic Heart Failure of the European Society of C, Bax JJ, Baumgartner H, Ceconi C, Dean V, Deaton C, Fagard R, Funck-Brentano C, Hasdai D, Hoes A, Kirchhof P, Knuuti J, Kolh P, McDonagh T, Moulin C, Popescu BA, Reiner Z, Sechtem U, Sirnes PA, Tendera M, Torbicki A, Vahanian A, Windecker S,

McDonagh T, Sechtem U, Bonet LA, Avraamides P, Ben Lamin HA, Brignole M, Coca A, Cowburn P, Dargie H, Elliott P, Flachskampf FA, Guida GF, Hardman S, Lung B, Merkely B, Mueller C, Nanas JN, Nielsen OW, Orn S, Parissis JT, Ponikowski P, Guidelines ESCCfP. ESC guidelines for the diagnosis and treatment of acute and chronic heart failure 2012: The Task Force for the Diagnosis and Treatment of Acute and Chronic Heart Failure 2012 of the European Society of Cardiology. Developed in collaboration with the Heart Failure Association (HFA) of the ESC. Eur J Heart Fail. 2012;14:803–69.

O'Connor DJ, Scher LA, Gargiulo 3rd NJ, Jang J, Suggs WD, Lipsitz EC. Incidence and characteristics of venous thromboembolic disease during pregnancy and the postnatal period: a contemporary series. Ann Vasc Surg. 2010;25(1):9–14.

Oran B, Lee-Parritz A, Ansell J. Low molecular weight heparin for the prophylaxis of thromboembolism in women with prosthetic mechanical heart valves during pregnancy. Thromb Haemost. 2004;92:747–51.

Quinn J, Von Klemperer K, Brooks R, Peebles D, Walker F, Cohen H. Use of high intensity adjusted dose low molecular weight heparin in women with mechanical heart valves during pregnancy: a single-center experience. Haematologica. 2009;94:1608–12.

Regitz-Zagrosek V, Blomstrom Lundqvist C, Borghi C, Cifkova R, Ferreira R, Foidart JM, Gibbs JS, Gohlke-Baerwolf C, Gorenek B, Iung B, Kirby M, Maas AH, Morais J, Nihoyannopoulos P, Pieper PG, Presbitero P, Roos-Hesselink JW, Schaufelberger M, Seeland U, Torracca L, Bax J, Auricchio A, Baumgartner H, Ceconi C, Dean V, Deaton C, Fagard R, Funck-Brentano C, Hasdai D, Hoes A, Knuuti J, Kolh P, McDonagh T, Moulin C, Poldermans D, Popescu BA, Reiner Z, Sechtem U, Sirnes PA, Torbicki A, Vahanian A, Windecker S, Aguiar C, Al-Attar N, Garcia AA, Antoniou A, Coman I, Elkayam U, Gomez-Sanchez MA, Gotcheva N, Hilfiker-Kleiner D, Kiss RG, Kitsiou A, Konings KT, Lip GY, Manolis A, Mebaaza A, Mintale I, Morice MC, Mulder BJ, Pasquet A, Price S, Priori SG, Salvador MJ, Shotan A, Silversides CK, Skouby SO, Stein JI, Tornos P, Vejlstrup N, Walker F, Warnes C. ESC guidelines on the management of cardiovascular diseases during pregnancy: the Task Force on the Management of Cardiovascular Diseases during Pregnancy of the European Society of Cardiology (ESC). Eur Heart J. 2011;32:3147–97.

Roth A, Elkayam U. Acute myocardial infarction associated with pregnancy. J Am Coll Cardiol. 2008;52:171–80.

Royal College of Obstetricians and Gynecologists. Reducing the risk of thrombosis and embolism during pregnancy and the puerperium, Green-top guideline No.37a. London: RCOG; 2009.

Rutherford SE, Phelan JP. Deep venous thrombosis and pulmonary embolism in pregnancy. Obstet Gynecol Clin North Am. 1991;18:345–70.

Schaefer C, Hannemann D, Meister R, Elefant E, Paulus W, Vial T, Reuvers M, Robert-Gnansia E, Arnon J, De Santis M, Clementi M, Rodriguez-Pinilla E, Dolivo A, Merlob P. Vitamin K antagonists and pregnancy outcome. A multi-centre prospective study. Thromb Haemost. 2006;95:949–57.

Sillesen M, Hjortdal V, Vejlstrup N, Sorensen K. Pregnancy with prosthetic heart valves – 30 years' nationwide experience in Denmark. Eur J Cardiothorac Surg. 2011;40(2):448–54.

Sliwa K, Hilfiker-Kleiner D, Petrie MC, Mebazaa A, Pieske B, Buchmann E, Regitz-Zagrosek V, Schaufelberger M, Tavazzi L, van Veldhuisen DJ, Watkins H, Shah AJ, Seferovic PM, Elkayam U, Pankuweit S, Papp Z, Mouquet F, McMurray JJ. Current state of knowledge on aetiology, diagnosis, management, and therapy of peripartum cardiomyopathy: a position statement from the Heart Failure Association of the European Society of Cardiology Working Group on peripartum cardiomyopathy. Eur J Heart Fail. 2010;12:767–78.

Sullivan EA, Ford JB, Chambers G, Slaytor EK. Maternal mortality in Australia, 1973-1996. Aust N Z J Obstet Gynaecol. 2004;44:452–7; discussion 377.

Torbicki A, Perrier A, Konstantinides S, Agnelli G, Galie N, Pruszczyk P, Bengel F, Brady AJ, Ferreira D, Janssens U, Klepetko W, Mayer E, Remy-Jardin M, Bassand JP, Vahanian A, Camm J, De Caterina R, Dean V, Dickstein K, Filippatos G, Funck-Brentano C, Hellemans I, Kristensen SD, McGregor K, Sechtem U, Silber S, Tendera M, Widimsky P, Zamorano JL, Zamorano JL, Andreotti F, Ascherman M, Athanassopoulos G, De Sutter J, Fitzmaurice D, Forster T, Heras M, Jondeau G, Kjeldsen K, Knuuti J, Lang I, Lenzen M, Lopez-Sendon J, Nihoyannopoulos P, Perez Isla L, Schwehr U, Torraca L, Vachiery JL. Guidelines on the diagnosis and management of acute pulmonary embolism: the Task Force for the Diagnosis and Management of Acute Pulmonary Embolism of the European Society of Cardiology (ESC). Eur Heart J. 2008;29:2276–315.

Turrentine MA, Braems G, Ramirez MM. Use of thrombolytics for the treatment of thromboembolic disease during pregnancy. Obstet Gynecol Surv. 1995;50:534–41.

Vahanian A, Alfieri O, Andreotti F, Antunes MJ, Baron-Esquivias G, Baumgartner H, Borger MA, Carrel TP, De Bonis M, Evangelista A, Falk V, Lung B, Lancellotti P, Pierard L, Price S, Schafers HJ, Schuler G, Stepinska J, Swedberg K, Takkenberg J, Von Oppell U O, Windecker S, Zamorano JL, Zembala M, Guidelines ESCCfP, Joint Task Force on the Management of Valvular Heart Disease of the European Society of C, European Association for Cardio-Thoracic S. Guidelines on the management of valvular heart disease (version 2012): the Joint Task Force on the Management of Valvular Heart Disease of the European Society of Cardiology (ESC) and the European Association for Cardio-Thoracic Surgery (EACTS). Eur J Cardiothorac Surg. 2012;42:S1–44.

van Driel D, Wesseling J, Sauer PJ, Touwen BC, van der Veer E, Heymans HS. Teratogen update: fetal effects after in utero exposure to coumarins overview of cases, follow-up findings, and pathogenesis. Teratology. 2002;66:127–40.

Vitale N, De Feo M, De Santo LS, Pollice A, Tedesco N, Cotrufo M. Dose-dependent fetal complications of warfarin in pregnant women with mechanical heart valves. J Am Coll Cardiol. 1999;33:1637–41.

Wilkinson H, Trustees and Medical Advisers. Saving mothers' lives. Reviewing maternal deaths to make motherhood safer: 2006-2008. BJOG. 2011;118:1402–3; discussion 1403–4.

Winer-Muram HT, Boone JM, Brown HL, Jennings SG, Mabie WC, Lombardo GT. Pulmonary embolism in pregnant patients: fetal radiation dose with helical CT. Radiology. 2002;224:487–92.

Yinon Y, Siu SC, Warshafsky C, Maxwell C, McLeod A, Colman JM, Sermer M, Silversides CK. Use of low molecular weight heparin in pregnant women with mechanical heart valves. Am J Cardiol. 2009;104:1259–63.

Obstetric Drugs in the Management of Cardiovascular Disease

Catherine Elliott

Introduction

Cardiac Disease complicates 0.6 % of pregnancies in South Africa (Sliwa et al. 2010). The term cardiac disease encompasses all possible heart disease from structural congenital lesions, to functional abnormalities and acquired valve lesions. When women suffering from cardiac disease conceive, the physiological haemodynamic changes in pregnancy as well as potential obstetric complications can result in cardiac deterioration. Medications used in the management of both routine general obstetrics and in the case of obstetric emergencies may adversely affect the heart function. Knowledge of the mechanisms of action of obstetric medications and potential side effects is vital when managing pregnant women with heart disease.

This chapter will discuss the effect of drugs used in obstetric management on the cardiovascular system.

C. Elliott, MBChB, FCOG (SA), MMED (UCT)
Department of Obstetrics and Gynaecology, Groote Schuur Hospital, Observatory, Cape Town 7925, South Africa
e-mail: elliottcath@hotmail.com

K. Sliwa, J. Anthony (eds.), *Cardiac Drugs in Pregnancy*, 107
Current Cardiovascular Therapy,
DOI 10.1007/978-1-4471-5472-3_6,
© Springer-Verlag London 2014

The Physiological Changes in Pregnancy

The physiological adaptions in pregnancy, designed to support the pregnancy and placental perfusion include circulatory adaptions. These are usually well tolerated in pregnancy, but may adversely affect cardiac function in the presence of heart disease.

The central adaption is peripheral vasodilatation with a decrease in peripheral vascular resistance. Following this, the cardiac output increases by about 40–50 % mostly due to an increase in stroke volume and secondly due to an increase in the heart rate (10–20 beats/min) from about 60–80 bpm (Nelson-Piercy 2002). The blood pressure will decrease due to the drop in peripheral vascular resistance. There is a 40–50 % increase in blood volume and another 50 % increase at delivery when there is an autrotransfusion of blood from the contracting uterus into the general circulation (Powrie 2010; Elliott 2012).

These changes can occur as early as the first trimester, and usually return to baseline by 6 weeks postpartum (Powrie 2010). The normal heart can tolerate these changes well, and pregnancies remain uncomplicated, however in the case of heart disease, be it structural or functional, the circulatory system may be compromised. The stressors placed on the heart may put the mother at increased risk of a cardiac event and even death, and any decrease in cardiac output will reduce placental perfusion and result in potential fetal hypoxemia.

Medications Used in Obstetric Practice

Tocolytic Therapy

Tocolysis is the medical suppression of uterine contractions, with the aim of arresting labour in the case of preterm labour, or decreasing the intensity and frequency of contractions, in the case of fetal distress, in preparation for emergency caesarian section. Arresting labour in the case of preterm labour will allow for the administration of cortico-steroids both to promote fetal lung maturity and thereby reduce the risk of respiratory distress syndrome, and to reduce the risk of intraventricular haemorrhage in the pre-term neonate. Inhibiting uterine contractions allows for the transfer, in utero, of the fetus to a neonatal facility of the appropriate level of care and thereby reducing the risk of perinatal mortality. Tocolysis is therefore effective in improving perinatal outcome by prolonging pregnancy for 48 h, but is not of great value if used as maintenance therapy (Roos et al. 2013).

Commonly used tocolytics include β-agonists, calcium channel blockers, oxytocin receptor antagonists, prostaglan-din synthetase inhibitors, nitric oxide donors and magnesium sulphate (used in United States of America) (Royal College of Obstetrics and Gynaecology 2011).

β-agonists

These drugs stimulate the β-receptors (predominantly β_2 adrenergic receptors), which have the effect of relaxing smooth muscle in sites including the myometrium, arterioles and bronchioles. This is achieved by the drug binding to the β-receptor as it is structurally similar to that of the endoge-nous catecholamines (Caughey and Parer 2001). This results in the stimulation of adenylate cyclase on the uterine smooth muscle (Royal College of Obstetrics and Gynaecology 2011; Caughey and Parer 2001) and a cascade of reactions culmi-nating in the inhibition of myosin light chain kinase and the resultant relaxation of the smooth muscle (in this case the uterine myocyte) (Caughey and Parer 2001). This class of drug includes ritodrine hydrochloride, hexoprenaline (Ipradol®), terbutaline and salbutamol. In industrialized countries ritodrine was until fairly recently the drug of choice and was widely used. Ritodrine is effective in delaying delivery for 48 h, but not any more effective than placebo in prolonging the pregnancy to term (The Canadian Preterm Labor Investigators Group 1992).

The use of these drugs as first-line tocolytic treatment has decreased in recent years due to the associated adverse effects and the introduction of newer drugs.

β-agonists are administered as an IVI infusion or as bolus injection given slowly over 10 min. The half-life is 150 min. The parenteral administration of β agonists elicits undesirable side effects, which include haemodynamic effects such as a marked tachycardia and peripheral vasodilation (Romero et al. 2000). The rise in pulse rate is the most common side effect and can increase by as much as 30 bpm (Moutquin et al. 2000).

This is disadvantageous in any condition associated with reduced left ventricular filling. Stroke volume and cardiac output depends on ventricular filling. In lesions such as a tight mitral stenosis, or atrial fibrillation, the left ventricular filling is already suboptimal, and tachyarrhythmia is particularly dangerous (Nelson-Piercy 2002).

Ritodrine crosses the placenta and fetal concentrations have been reported to be anything from 20 to 100 % (Valenzuela et al. 1995). The tachycardia elicited by β-agonists, is often also reflected by the development of a fetal tachycardia (Moutquin et al. 2000).

Additional side effects have been listed and include maternal arrhythmias, nausea, palpitations, dyspnea (Caughey and Parer 2001) hyperglycemia, tremor, hypokalemia and altered thyroid function tests (Caughey and Parer 2001; The Canadian Preterm Labor Investigators Group 1992; Moutquin et al. 2000). A rare but significant side effect includes the onset of fulminant pulmonary edema, especially when β_2-agonists are used in conjunction with corticosteroids to promote fetal lung maturity or when used in the patient with heart disease (described in the setting of tight mitral stenosis) (The Canadian Preterm Labor Investigators Group 1992).

In summary, β_2-agonists are very effective in delaying delivery for 48 h thereby fulfilling the criteria for effective tocolysis, but are contraindicated in patients with heart disease.

Nifedipine

Nifedipine is a dihydropyridine calcium channel blocker. It is used in South Africa as a cost effective tocolytic. It is conveniently administered orally.

The efficacy of nifedipine is comparable to other standard tocolytics such as ritodrine as well as the newer drugs such as atosiban (see below) (Royal College of Obstetrics and Gynaecology, Kashanian et al. 2005). Calcium channel blockers limit the release of calcium from the sarcoplasmic reticulum and thereby decrease the contractility of muscle. The effect can be variable in pregnancy due to differing expression of the cytochrome P450 3A substrate. This enzyme is responsible for the metabolism of nifedipine, with the genotype carried by the patient influencing the oral clearance of the drug (David 2013).

The main side effect is that of hypotension (Kashanian et al. 2005). Other listed side effects include, tachycardia, flushing, headache, syncope, dizziness, palpitations and rarely cardiac failure (Kashanian et al. 2005). The side effect profile is considered to be better than that of the β_2-agonists (Royal College of Obstetrics and Gynaecology 2011) and is therefore often used in preference to the β_2-agonists.

The safety of nifedipine has been well established in the general population; however in the presence of heart disease its use can have severe consequences. Myocardial infarction, congestive cardiac failure and pulmonary edema have all been described with the administration of nifedipine as a tocolytic. These complications may be directly ascribed to the drug, rather than the underlying cardiac condition. The use of this drug is contraindicated in cases where there is comorbidity in the form of sepsis, cardiac disease, thyroid disease or any degree of hypovolemia. The cardiovascular effects of hypotension and resultant tachycardia preclude its use in patients with heart disease. It has been known to cause sudden death in pregnant patients with undiagnosed heart disease and should never be administered indiscriminately.

In summary, nifedipine is an effective tocolytic. Oral administration is convenient. However, it should not be administered without full knowledge of any underlying comorbidity.

Atosiban

Atosiban is a nona-peptide oxytocin analog that acts as a competitive, selective oxytocin vasopressin receptor antagonist and inhibits oxytocin induced uterine contractions and is used as a tocolytic (Romero et al. 2000; Moutquin et al. 2000; Kashanian et al. 2005; Goodwin et al. 1995).

Atosiban is administered as an intravenous infusion. It has a half-life of 20 min and therefore plasma levels decrease rapidly after cessation of administration (Valenzuela et al. 1995; Kashanian et al. 2005).

This half-life means that a steady state is achieved fairly quickly, (within 1 h of administration) (Goodwin et al. 1995). Atosiban has been found to be effective in delaying delivery by 48 h in the case of preterm labour (Valenzuela et al. 2000).

Maintenance therapy using atosiban is also effective in maintaining uterine quiescence, and can be administered as a subcutaneous infusion. The safety profile of atosiban is at least comparable and possibly better than that of β_2-agonists (Valenzuela et al. 2000), although some patients choose to discontinue the drug due to drip-site inflammation and irritation.

The efficacy of Atosiban has been found to be the same as other standard tocolytics mentioned above, namely, ritodrine and nifedipine, however the side effects are much reduced, and do not compare to those associated with the β_2-agonists or calcium channel blockers (Kashanian et al. 2005; Moutquin et al. 2000). Atosiban is therefore, not contraindicated in cardiac patients (Royal College of Obstetrics and Gynaecology 2011) and the benefit of using atosiban lies - in the improved maternal side effect profile. Listed side effects include nausea, vomiting and chest pain, although the latter has not been found to occur more frequently than placebo, In particular, studies have shown there is a negligible incidence of tachycardia and chest pain and cardiovascular side-effects are substantially lower than those associated with the use of ritodrine (Moutquin et al. 2000). In fact, when compared to placebo, atosiban showed no significant differences in side-effect profile and women undergoing tocolysis do not discontinue atosiban due to side effects, as they do with ritodrine (Romero et al. 2000; Valenzuela et al. 2000).

In addition, the use of atosiban produced no cases of pulmonary edema when compared to placebo (Romero et al. 2000). Atosiban does not appear to cross the placenta and does not accumulate in the fetal circulation.

In summary, Atosiban has been recommended as the tocolytic of choice when managing preterm labour in patients with heart disease (Kashanian et al. 2005).

Non-steroidal Anti-inflammatory Drugs

Cox-2 inhibitors, inhibit the production of prostaglandins, and are used before 32 weeks gestation as a tocolytic (Gibbon 2005). Indomethacin inhibits the cyclooxygenase enzyme in the conversion of arachydonic acid to prostaglandins. Prostaglandins increase the intracellular calcium in the uterine myocyte (Vermillion and Landen 2001) and are also implicated in the cervical changes occurring at the onset of labour both at term and preterm gestations. Premature closure of the ductus arteriosus has been found in the fetus if used after this gestation, although some authors would suggest that this risk has been exaggerated (Nelson-Piercy 2002). The most commonly used drug from this class is indomethacin (Indocid®), which is usually administered orally, but may also be given per rectum (Vermillion and Landen 2001). Cox-2 inhibitors are contraindicated in the case of ischemic heart disease (IHD) and in patients who have a high risk of IHD. They cause an increase in peripheral vascular resistance (Sorensen et al. 1992), (although the blood pressure may not change) and have been associated with an increased risk of adverse cardiac events, such as myocardial infarction (Nelson-Piercy 2002; Gibbon 2005) and should be used with caution in hypertensive patients (Sorensen et al. 1992).

Magnesium Sulphate

The use of magnesium sulphate as a tocolytic is confined in most part to the United States of America. It is mentioned here to complete the list of tocolytics. The mechanism of action of magnesium sulphate as a tocolytic is not fully understood (Ramsey and Rouse 2001), and the Cochrane Collaboration disputes this indication. Those in favour of its tocolytic potential, suggest administering it as a loading dose and then as an infusion to maintain levels of 5–8 mg/dL which will allow for a therapeutic decrease in muscular contractility, including in the myocyte. Toxicity may lead to maternal respiratory failure due to intercostal muscle paralysis (Ramsey and Rouse 2001). It is excreted by the kidneys and absolute contraindications are myasthenia gravis and heart block (Ramsey and Rouse 2001). Apart from a mild drop in blood pressure, magnesium sulphate does not have any major effects on the cardiovascular system.

Oxytocic Therapy

These drugs enhance uterine contractions and are used to augment labour, induce labour or to terminate a pregnancy.

They are also used postpartum in the management of the third stage of labour and in the management of postpartum haemorrhage to facilitate uterine contraction.

These drugs include: oxytocin, ergometrine and the prostaglandins, F_2alpha and misoprostol.

Oxytocin

Oxytocin is a polypeptide hormone, which has been artificially synthesized (Dyer et al. 2010). By binding to the surface of the uterine myocyte, oxytocin results in the synthesis of prostaglandin via the generation of diacylglycerol (DAG), inositol tri-phosphate and via the COX-2 pathway as well as by triggering the release of calcium from the sarcoplasmic reticulum. This results in contraction of the myometrial smooth muscle. When oxytocin is administered as a rate controlled infusion, the myometrial response is contraction followed by relaxation in a cyclical fashion (Gohil 2001) This drug is used for the induction or augmentation of labour. When used in this clinical setting, it is administered as an IVI infusion via an infusion pump and the rate is titrated against uterine contractions. This formulation of oxytocin is fast acting (within 5 min) and the effect lasts up to 1 h, however a rapid decrease in response is seen in the first 10 min after discontinuation. The half-life is 3 min (Gibbon 2005).

Oxytocin is also administered as a once off intramuscular injection directly after the delivery of the placenta to provoke uterine contraction as part of the active management of the third stage of labour. At caesarean section, it is given as a slow intravenous bolus of 5 IU for the same indication. Active management of the third stage of labour reduces the risk of post-partum haemorrhage by ensuring the early delivery of the separated placenta.

Oxytocin should be used judiciously in the induction or augmentation of labour. Complications of the administration include uterine hyperstimulation and resultant fetal distress. Careful monitoring of the effect in terms of frequency and amplitude of uterine contractions is mandatory, as is regular, if not continuous fetal heart rate monitoring.

During the administration of oxytocin, pulmonary wedge pressure is markedly increased. A rare but serious complication is hyponatraemia with cerebral edema and convulsions have been described with high doses, as oxytocin has a similar structure to that of vasopressin (Gibbon 2005; Dyer et al. 2010).

The haemodynamic effects of oxytocin are not well tolerated in patients with poor ventricular function, or in those where a decrease in peripheral vascular resistance will worsen the clinical scenario, such as in the case of stenotic heart lesions, or those who have poor ventricular function due to cardiomyopathy. This drug is used with caution in patients with cardiac disease and some authors will state that it is in fact contraindicated in patients with heart disease.

Ergometrine

This medication belongs to the class of ergot alkaloids (www.mims.com/USA/drug/info/ergometrine) and is usually administered in the management of obstetric haemorrhage caused by uterine atony.

It is administered by intravenous injection as a bolus dose; it may be administered up to four times a day for 48 h and has an immediate onset of action (Gohil 2001).

Ergometrine causes rapid contraction of the uterine muscle, which is sustained over time. In low doses, an increase in frequency and amplitude of the contractions is noted while high doses, result in an increase in uterine tone (www.mms.com/USA/drug/info/ergometrine). The mechanism of action is not fully understood. Due to these effects, ergometrine is never used prior to delivery of the fetus.

Ergometrine has a half-life of 2 h. The side effects associated with the use of ergometrine include breathing difficulties, chest pain, dizziness, headaches, palpitations, and arrhythmias, raised blood pressure, vasoconstriction, vomiting and pulmonary edema.

Although oxytocin is used as the first-line agent for treating postpartum haemorrhage, ergometrine has been found to be a very effective oxytocic drug, and in fact superior, to other oxytocics such as oxytocin (Aflaifel and Weeks 2012). Unless ergometrine is contraindicated the benefits of its use outweigh the risks in the setting of ongoing uterine atony despite oxytocin administration (Aflaifel and Weeks 2012).

Ergometrine is contraindicated in the case of cardiac disease, due to the vasoconstrictive effects. It causes vasoconstriction in the peripheral and cerebral vessels, leading to an 11 % increase in mean arterial blood pressure (Dyer et al. 2010) and a 30 % increase in pulmonary artery pressure (Dyer et al. 2010). It can also cause spasm of the renal arteries and the coronary arteries, resulting in myocardial infarction in rare cases (Dyer et al. 2010).

Syntometrine is the combination of oxytocin and ergometrine (5 IU oxytocin and 0.5 mg ergometrine) and is administered as a single IMI dose in the active management of the third stage of labour, and occasionally it is used as a single dose given to prevent postpartum haemorrhage in high-risk cases. In this combination, the oxytocin ensures a rapid onset of oxytocic action while the ergometrine ensures that the oxytocic effect lasts for several hours (Dyer et al. 2010). However, this formulation causes a marked elevation in blood pressure and commonly results in nausea and vomiting.

Prostaglandins

Prostaglandins increase the calcium concentration inside the myocyte via G-protein (Dyer et al. 2010). Prostaglandins provoke and enhance uterine contractions, and are used in the treatment of severe postpartum haemorrhage as a third line agent. $PGF_2\alpha$ is the prostaglandin used for this indication. It is administered intramuscularly, directly into the myometrium, either under direct vision at the time of caesarean laparotomy or via the anterior abdominal wall using a long needle. Inadvertent intravascular administration of $PGF_2\alpha$ may cause severe bronchospasm leading to hypoxemia. Marked hypertension and pulmonary hypertension are also likely consequences of intravenous injection.

Misoprostol

Misoprostol is a 16-methyl prostaglandin E_1 analogue and is a relatively low cost medication. It is used off label for the induction of labour, termination of pregnancy and in the management of postpartum haemorrhage due to uterine atony. In this setting it is usually used only as a first line agent when others are unavailable, such as in the setting of a home birth. Misoprostol does not need to be kept in the fridge. It can be administered orally, sublingually, rectally and vaginally. If it is administered vaginally it has not been found to have any haemodynamic effect (Dyer et al. 2010).

Magnesium Sulphate for Neuroprotection

Magnesium sulphate is administered antenatally to a mother at risk of preterm delivery at less than 30 weeks gestation, for its beneficial effect on the fetus. It has a neuroprotective effect on the fetal brain and has been shown to decrease the risk of severe gross motor dysfunction and cerebral palsy in the preterm neonate and children up to 2 years (Doyle 2010; Crowther et al. 2003). It is administered as a loading bolus via an infusion of 6 g followed by a continuous infusion of 2 g/h (Rouse et al. 2008). Magnesium sulphate is predominantly excreted by the renal system and maternal urine output must remain at a minimum of 30 ml/h. Magnesium sulphate has not been shown to have any major effects on the maternal cardiovascular system. In its use in this setting has not demonstrated any adverse maternal complications.

TABLE 1 Medications used in obstetric practice and their cardiovascular effects

Medication	Example	Indication	Main adverse effects on the cardiovascular system
β-agonists	Hexoprenaline (Ipradol)®	Tocolysis	Tachycardia
			Peripheral vasodilatation
			Pulmonary edema
Calcium channel blocker	Nifedipine (Adalat®)	Tocolysis	Hypotension
		Hypertension	Tachycardia
Oxytocin receptor antagonist	Atosiban (Antocin®)	Tocolysis	None
NSAIDs	Indomethacin (Indocid®)	Tocolysis	Vasoconstriction
MgSO4	MgSO4	Neuroprotection for the fetus Tocolysis in USA	Almost none
Oxytocin	Oxytocin (Syntocinon®)	Labour augmentation or induction Uterine involution	Hypotension
Ergot alkaloids	Ergometrine (Ergometrine®)	Postpartum haemorrhage	Vasoconstriction
Prostaglandins F₂Alpha	Dinoprost (Prostin F₂Alpha®)	Postpartum haemorrhage/TOP	Bronchospasm
Prostaglandin E₁	Misoprostol (Cytotec®)	Induction of labour/TOP Postpartum haemorrhage	None

Conclusion

Almost all medications used in obstetric practice have cardiovascular effects. The use of drugs with potential adverse effects on the cardiovascular system may increase the likelihood of morbidity and mortality in pregnant women with heart disease. A thorough knowledge of the patient's current and prior medical history is mandatory before administering any medication, and medications known to have haemodynamic consequences are best avoided in patients with known cardiac disease.

References

Aflaifel N, Weeks AD. Active management of the third stage of labour. BMJ. 2012;345:e4546.

Caughey AB, Parer JT. Tocolysis with beta-adrenergic receptor agonists. Semin Perinatol. 2001;25:248–55.

Crowther CA, Hiller JE, Doyle LW, Haslam RR, Australasian Collaborative Trial of Magnesium Sulphate Collaborative Group. Effect of magnesium sulfate given for neuroprotection before preterm birth: a randomized controlled trial. JAMA. 2003;290:2669–76.

David M. Nifedipine pharmacokinetics are influenced by the CYP. Am J Perinatol. 2013;30:275–82.

Doyle L. Magnesium sulphate for women at risk of preterm birth for neuroprotection of the fetus. Cochrane Database Syst Rev. 2010;(3):CD004661. http://www.thecochranelibrary.com.

Dyer RA, van Dyk D, Dresner A. The use of uterotonic drugs during caesarean section. Int J Obstet Anesth. 2010;19:313–9.

Elliott C. Complications of anticoagulation on the management of pregnant women with mechanical heart valves. MMED, University of Cape Town, 2012.

Gibbon C. South African medical formulary. 7th ed. Cape Town: South African Medical Association; 2005.

Gohil T. A study to compare the efficacy of misoprostol, oxytocin, methyl-ergometrine and ergometrin-oxytocin in reducing blood loss in active management of 3rd stage of labour. J Obstet Gynaecol India. 2001;61:408–12.

Goodwin TM, Millar L, North L, Abrams LS, Weglein RC, Holland ML. The pharmacokinetics of the oxytocin antagonist atosiban in pregnant women with preterm uterine contractions. Am J Obstet Gynecol. 1995;173:913–7.

Kashanian M, Akbarian AR, Soltanzadeh M. Atosiban and nifedipin for the treatment of preterm labor. Int J Gynaecol Obstet. 2005;91:10–4.

Moutquin JM, Sherman D, Cohen H, Mohide PT, Hochner-Celnikier D, Fejgin M, Liston RM, Dansereau J, Mazor M, Shalev E, Boucher M, Glezerman M, Zimmer EZ, Rabinovici J. Double-blind, randomized, controlled trial of atosiban and ritodrine in the treatment of preterm labor: a multicenter effectiveness and safety study. Am J Obstet Gynecol. 2000;182:1191–9.

Nelson-Piercy C. Medical disorders of pregnancy. 4th ed. New York: Informa Healthcare; 2002.

Powrie R. De Swiet's medical disorders in obstetric practice. 5th ed. Chichester: Wiley-Blackwell; 2010.

Ramsey PS, Rouse DJ. Magnesium sulfate as a tocolytic agent. Semin Perinatol. 2001;25:236–47.

Romero R, Sibai BM, Sanchez-Ramos L, Valenzuela GJ, Veille JC, Tabor B, Perry KG, Varner M, Goodwin TM, Lane R, Smith J, Shangold G, Creasy GW. An oxytocin receptor antagonist (atosiban) in the treatment of preterm labor: a randomized, double-blind, placebo-controlled trial with tocolytic rescue. Am J Obstet Gynecol. 2000;182:1173–83.

Roos C, Spaanderman ME, Schuit E, Bloemenkamp KW, Bolte AC, Cornette J, Duvekot JJ, van Eyck J, Franssen MT, de Groot CJ, Kok JH, Kwee A, Merien A, Nij Bijvank B, Opmeer BC, Oudijk MA, van Pampus MG, Papatsonis DN, Porath MM, Scheepers HC, Scherjon SA, Sollie KM, Vijgen SM, Willekes C, Mol BW, van der Post JA, Lotgering FK, APOSTEL-II Study Group. Effect of maintenance tocolysis with nifedipine in threatened preterm labor on perinatal outcomes: a randomized controlled trial. JAMA. 2013;309:41–7.

Rouse DJ, Hirtz DG, Thom E, Varner MW, Spong CY, Mercer BM, Iams JD, Wapner RJ, Sorokin Y, Alexander JM, Harper M, Thorp Jr JM, Ramin SM, Malone FD, Carpenter M, Miodovnik M, Moawad A, O'Sullivan MJ, Peaceman AM, Hankins GD, Langer O, Caritis SN, Roberts JM, Eunice Kennedy Shriver, N. M.-F. M. U. N. A randomized, controlled trial of magnesium sulfate for the prevention of cerebral palsy. N Engl J Med. 2008;359:895–905.

Royal College of Obstetrics and Gynaecology. Tocolysis for women in preterm labour. London: Royal College of Obstetrics and Gynaecology; 2011. http://www.rcog.org.uk/womens-health/clinical-guidance/tocolytic-drugs-women-preterm-labour-green-top-1b.

Sliwa K, Hilfiker-Kleiner D, Petrie M, Mebazaa A, Pieske B, Buchmann E, Regitz-Zagrosek V, Schaufelberger M, Tavazzi B, van Veldhuisen DJ, Watkins H, Shah AJ, Seferovic PM, Elkayam U, Pankuweit S, Papp Z, Mouquet F, McMurray J. Current state of knowledge on aetiology, diagnosis, management, and therapy of peripartum cardiomyopathy: a position statement from the Heart Failure Association of the European Society of Cardiology Working Group on Peripartum Cardiomyopathy. Eur Heart J. 2010;12:767–78.

Sorensen TK, Easterling TR, Carlson KL, Brateng DA, Benedetti TJ. The maternal hemodynamic effect of indomethacin in normal pregnancy. Obstet Gynecol. 1992;79:661–3.

The Canadian Preterm Labor Investigators Group. Treatment of preterm labor with the beta-adrenergic agonist ritodrine. N Engl J Med. 1992;327:308–12.

Valenzuela GJ, Craig J, Bernhardt MD, Holland ML. Placental passage of the oxytocin antagonist atosiban. Am J Obstet Gynecol. 1995;172: 1304–6.

Valenzuela GJ, Sanchez-Ramos L, Romero R, Silver HM, Koltun WD, Millar L, Hobbins J, Rayburn W, Shangold G, Wang J, Smith J, Creasy GW. Maintenance treatment of preterm labor with the oxytocin antagonist atosiban. The Atosiban PTL-098 Study Group. Am J Obstet Gynecol. 2000;182:1184–90.

Vermillion ST, Landen CN. Prostaglandin inhibitors as tocolytic agents. Semin Perinatol. 2001;25:256–62.

Index

K. Sliwa, J. Anthony (eds.), *Cardiac Drugs in Pregnancy*,
Current Cardiovascular Therapy,
DOI 10.1007/978-1-4471-5472-3,
© Springer-Verlag London 2014